CARDIOLOGY RESEARCH AND CLINICAL DEVELOPMENTS

CURRENT ISSUES IN THE MANAGEMENT OF STABLE ISCHEMIC HEART DISEASE

CARDIOLOGY RESEARCH AND CLINICAL DEVELOPMENTS

Additional books in this series can be found on Nova's website
under the Series tab.

Additional e-books in this series can be found on Nova's website
under the e-book tab.

CARDIOLOGY RESEARCH AND CLINICAL DEVELOPMENTS

CURRENT ISSUES IN THE MANAGEMENT OF STABLE ISCHEMIC HEART DISEASE

MUKESH SINGH
EDITOR

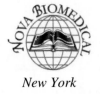

New York

NOTICE TO THE READER

The Publisher has taken reasonable care in the preparation of this book, but makes no expressed or implied warranty of any kind and assumes no responsibility for any errors or omissions. No liability is assumed for incidental or consequential damages in connection with or arising out of information contained in this book. The Publisher shall not be liable for any special, consequential, or exemplary damages resulting, in whole or in part, from the readers' use of, or reliance upon, this material. Any parts of this book based on government reports are so indicated and copyright is claimed for those parts to the extent applicable to compilations of such works.

Independent verification should be sought for any data, advice or recommendations contained in this book. In addition, no responsibility is assumed by the publisher for any injury and/or damage to persons or property arising from any methods, products, instructions, ideas or otherwise contained in this publication.

This publication is designed to provide accurate and authoritative information with regard to the subject matter covered herein. It is sold with the clear understanding that the Publisher is not engaged in rendering legal or any other professional services. If legal or any other expert assistance is required, the services of a competent person should be sought. FROM A DECLARATION OF PARTICIPANTS JOINTLY ADOPTED BY A COMMITTEE OF THE AMERICAN BAR ASSOCIATION AND A COMMITTEE OF PUBLISHERS.

Additional color graphics may be available in the e-book version of this book.

Library of Congress Cataloging-in-Publication Data

ISBN: 978-1-62417-203-8

Library of Congress Control Number: 2012951006

Published by Nova Science Publishers, Inc. † New York

Contents

Preface

Over the last four decades great strides have been made in reducing death from cardiovascular diseases. However, coronary artery disease (CAD) remains a significant source of morbidity and mortality in the United States as well as the world. It is estimated that 13,200,000 Americans have CAD, 6,500,000 of whom have angina pectoris with 400,000 new cases yearly. In the past two decades there has been extensive development in the field with better understanding of pathophysiology, the increased use of imaging modalities, development and availability of newer medications and revascularization techniques. As a consequence of this rapid development it has been difficult for practicing physicians to keep up-to-date with the innovations in this field. Management paradigms for treating angina revolve around reducing symptoms related to ischemia and preventing myocardial infarction or sudden cardiac death. Traditional options for CAD treatment include medical therapy and coronary revascularization. This volume is intended to be clear and concise in order to provide up to date understanding of the pathophysiology and management of stable ischemic heart disease. It illustrates the basic concepts related to evaluation and management of SIHD in easy to understand manner and reflects the key issues relevant to practicing cardiologists and internists in their care of patients. It encompasses the discussion of full spectrum of SIHD from clinical evaluation and management of chronic stable angina to refractory angina, microvascular angina and hibernating myocardium. It delineates the practical approach for evaluation and management of SIHD. It is our hope that cardiologists, in private practice and in academic medical centers, and physicians in training will benefit from the many illustrations and overall design of this book. It provides a rapid guide and reference to a broad spectrum of SIHD and the practice based approach should make it particularly valuable to practicing as well as in training physicians.

Mukesh Singh
Department of Cardiology
Mt. Sinai Hospital Medical Center,
Chicago, IL, US

In: Current Issues in the Management of Stable Ischemic Heart … ISBN: 978-1-62417-203-8
Editor: Mukesh Singh   © 2013 Nova Science Publishers, Inc.

Chapter I

Clinical Evaluation and Differential Diagnosis of Chest Pain

Jayanth Koneru[*], *Susan Phung,*
Oday Alrabadi and Mahesh Bikkina
St. Joseph Hospital, Paterson, New Jersey, US

Abstract

Angina pectoris, commonly referred to as angina, is chest pain due to ischemia of the cardiac muscle, secondary to obstruction or spasm of the coronary arteries.

Chest pain encompasses a vast spectrum of clinical etiologies which require thorough evaluation of the patient. Angina occurs when myocardial oxygen demand exceeds oxygen supply.

Classification of angina can be divided into stable angina, and unstable angina. This chapter will discuss in detail the symptoms, mechanism and differential diagnosis of angina, with brief outline of treatment of stable angina.

Introduction

Angina pectoris, commonly referred to as angina, is chest pain due to ischemia of the cardiac muscle, secondary to obstruction or spasm of the coronary arteries. Chest pain encompasses a vast spectrum of clinical etiologies which require thorough evaluation of the patient. A detailed differential diagnosis of patients presenting with chest pain from benign musculoskeletal etiologies to life-threatening cardiac disease will be discussed. Etiologies causing chest pain will be discussed in order of prevalence seen in primary care setting.

[*] Address for correspondence: Jayanth Koneru, MD; St. Joseph Regional Medical Center; 703 Main Street, Paterson, NJ 07503; United States; Phone: (248) 977-0987; Fax: 973-754-2327; Email: koneru. jayanth@gmail.com.

Angina occurs when myocardial oxygen demand exceeds oxygen supply. Classification of angina can be divided into stable angina, and unstable angina. This chapter will discuss in detail the symptoms, mechanism and differential diagnosis of angina, with brief outline of treatment of stable angina.

Differential Diagnosis of Chest Pain

Chest pain is one of the most common challenges for clinicians. The differential diagnosis includes conditions affecting organs within the thorax and abdomen, with prognostic implications that vary from relatively benign to requiring immediate medical intervention. Serious consequences, including death, can result from a failure to differentiate emergent conditions such as acute ischemic heart disease, aortic dissection, tension pneumothorax, and pulmonary embolism. On the other hand, defensive medical management of low risk patients can lead to unnecessary hospital admissions, prolonged hospital stay, and excessive diagnostic tests and procedures. The nature of the chest pain can be subsequently categorized into potentially life threatening conditions that warrant immediate hospitalization and aggressive evaluation, chronic conditions that can lead to serious complications, acute conditions that require specific treatment, and lastly conditions that have a more benign course. Cardiac causes of chest discomfort are frequently attributed, but not limited to myocardial ischemia and injury [1].

Myocardial ischemia occurs when the oxygen supply to the heart is not sufficient to meet the metabolic demands. This mismatch can result from a decrease in oxygen supply, an increase in demand, or both. Coronary artery disease remains one of the leading and most serious causes of chest discomfort [2,3].

Differential Diagnosis of Chest Pain

Cardiac	Pulmonary	Gastrointestinal	Miscellaneous
Coronary heart disease	Acute pulmonary embolism	Gastroesophageal Reflux Disease	Musculoskeletal Pain
Aortic Dissection	Pulmonary hypertension	Esophageal Hyperalgesia	Rheumatic Diseases
Valvular heart disease	Lung Parenchyma -Pneumonia -Malignancy -Sarcoidosis	Esophageal rupture	Psychogenic/Psychoso matic
Pericarditis	Pleura -Pneumothorax -Pleuritis -Pleural effusion	Medication induced esophagitis	
Myocarditis	Mediastinal Disease	Mediastinitis	
Stress induced cardiomyopathy			
Syndrome X			

The obstruction of coronary arteries by atherosclerosis can lead to a wide range of presentations of ischemic heart disease including stable angina to unstable angina, non-ST elevation myocardial infarction, and ST elevation myocardial infarction. As mentioned, patients with acute coronary syndrome often complain of chest heaviness, pressure, tightness, or burning that is associated with symptoms such as shortness of breath, palpitations, light headedness diaphoresis, nausea, or vomiting. Stable angina pectoris, in particular, generally develops gradually with exertion, emotional stress, or after heavy meals. Unstable angina, on the other hand, presents in a similar fashion to stable angina, but is more prolonged and severe. Whereas ST elevation MI requires immediate revascularization intervention, non-ST elevation MI can be further stratified into early invasive versus conservative strategies depending on patient risk factors [3].

Other major cardiac causes aside from ischemic heart disease include abnormalities of various structures such as the valves, the pericardium, or the great vessels. While severe mitral stenosis may be a cause of intermittent chest pain, the most common valvular lesion associated with progressive angina or dyspnea is severe aortic stenosis [2]. Signs of congestive heart failure or syncope in these patients tend to carry a grave prognosis. In conjunction with the valvular structures, inflammation of the pericardium, whether it is from one of numerous causes including infectious etiology, uremia, recent myocardial infarction, can present with chest pain. Although, the pain is believed to be due to the inflammation of the adjacent parietal pleura as most of the sensory innervation supplies the parietal pleura not the pericardium [4]. Classically, chest pain secondary to pericarditis is retrosternal, aggravated by coughing, deep inspiration, and is often positional. Rare cardiac cause of chest pain such as spontaneous coronary artery dissection, hypertrophic cardiomyopathy, and syndrome X should also be in the differential if the index of suspicion is high [5-7].

Diseases of the aorta, specifically aortic dissection is a diagnosis that should not be overlooked as the consequences could be detrimental. The pathophysiology of aortic dissection involves the tearing of the intima or the aorta or with rupture of the vasa vasorum within the media leading to the spread of a subintimal hematoma within the wall of the aorta with creation of a false lumen [8]. The predisposing factors for aortic dissection are varied, ranging from trauma, especially from motor vehicle accident, to iatrogenic procedures such as intra-aortic balloon pumps, to cystic medial degeneration secondary to connective tissue diseases such as Marfan's or Ehler-Danlos syndromes, to inflammatory diseases that cause vasculitis. However, the single most important risk factor for aortic dissection is systemic hypertension [8]. The clinical manifestation of aortic dissection is dependent upon the location of the extension of the dissection and the degree of compromise to blood flow in the branches of the aorta. For instance, patients often present with acute, sharp, "tearing" pain that radiates to the back, but involvement of the ascending aorta can result in acute aortic regurgitation, acute myocardial infarction, cardiac tamponade, or even cerebrovascular accident if there is extension into the carotid arteries. Moreover, extension into the descending aortic can cause paraplegia through ischemia of the spinal cord [2,3].

In addition to cardiac causes, gastrointestinal causes of chest pain are also quite common. Because the heart and esophagus share similar innervation, it is oftentimes difficult to distinguish between myocardial ischemia and symptoms originating from the gastrointestinal tract via clinical history alone. Moreover, the response of the chest discomfort to what is commonly referred to as the "GI cocktail", consisting of viscous lidocaine, liquid antacid, and an anticholinergic, does not aid in differentiating the two diagnoses as myocardial ischemia and dyspepsia may coexist. There are, however, features that are found more frequently in patients with esophageal chest discomfort. For instance, pain provoked by swallowing, postural changes, or associated with heartburn and regurgitation of acid into the mouth and alleviated by antacids is more suggestive of a gastrointestinal etiology. Other clues that point to esophageal origin include nocturnal pain, frequent episodes of spontaneous pain without radiation, and an inconsistent relationship to exercise.

Gastrointestinal causes of chest discomfort also vary tremendously from chronic conditions to highly acute conditions. Gastroesophageal reflux disease, in particular, can closely resemble the symptomatology of angina pectoris with a squeezing or burning substernal pain that can radiate to the back, jaw, neck, or arms [2]. Less common causes of chest discomfort such as esophageal hyperalgesia and motility disorders or esophageal spasm should be considered if the pain is associated with dysphagia. Even rarer conditions such as esophageal rupture with spontaneous perforation induced by either ingestion of caustic material, pill esophagitis, Barrett's ulcer, infectious ulcer, or iatrogenic injury should not be excluded from the differential as they require immediate medical intervention. More specifically, patients with medication induced esophagitis typically present with sudden onset of odynophagia and retrosternal pain that began with the onset of swallowing a pill without water. Medications that are known to cause direct esophageal injury are antibiotics, particularly doxycycline, anti-inflammatory agents, and bisphosphonates [2,3]. Aside from esophageal chest discomfort, it is also important to include referred visceral pain due to cholecystitis, peptic ulcer disease, biliary colic, pancreatitis, nephrolithiasis, and appendicitis in the differential.

Pulmonary etiologies of chest pain, similar to gastrointestinal etiologies, can be an acute condition such as pulmonary embolism or a chronic condition such as pulmonary hypertension. The pleura, the pulmonary vessels, as well as the lung parenchyma could be the source of the pain. Chest pain due to pulmonary embolism may be due to the distention of the pulmonary artery or infarction of a segment of the lung adjacent to the pleura. While a massive pulmonary embolus can lead to substernal pain resembling that of an acute myocardial infarction, acute pulmonary embolism often presents as smaller emboli that cause focal pulmonary infarctions resulting in a more pleuritic type of pain associated with dyspnea, tachycardia, and hemoptysis [9]. The patients who present with acute pulmonary embolism usually have risk factors such as immobilization, recent surgery, prior venous thromboembolism, hypercoaguable disorders, or malignancy. Like acute pulmonary embolism, spontaneous pneumothorax is another diagnosis that can be potentially lethal if missed. Typically, the patient complains of a sudden onset of pleuritic chest pain and respiratory distress, sometimes with underlying chronic obstructive pulmonary disease [10]. Tension pneumothorax progressively traps air in the intrapleural space during inspiration until the healthy lung becomes compressed and prompt decompression with a large bore needle is necessary. Diseases of the lung parenchyma such as pneumonia, malignancy, and rarely sarcoidosis should also be included in the differential. The pleura and pleural space can cause pleuritic chest pain via irritation of the nerve endings in the costal pleura, for example in autoimmune diseases such as systemic lupus erythematosus or rheumatoid arthritis.

Chest wall pain is yet another common cause of chest discomfort. Many times the chest wall pain is caused by musculoskeletal inflammation or costochondritis is associated with trauma or repetitive activity involving the upper trunk or arms. The presentation is often insidious, persistent, and localizes to a specific area or muscle group. Post herpetic neuralgia secondary to herpes zoster infection or postradiation neuralgia may also present as chest pain. Despite a history that is characteristic for chest wall pain, it is important to realize that musculoskeletal pain does not exclude the concomitant diagnosis of chest pain secondary to myocardial ischemia. Lastly, having ruled out all the organic and more gravid causes, consideration should be given to psychogenic and psychosomatic causes of chest pain. Chest pain may be a presenting syndrome of panic disorder, depression, hypochondriasis, Munchausen's syndrome, and other nonspecific phobias, just to name a few [11].

While the origin of chest discomfort is vast, the approach to the patient with this presentation requires a great degree of prudence. Etiologies such as acute myocardial infarction, pneumothorax, spontaneous pulmonary embolism should be quickly differentiated and treated, whereas other diagnoses including gastrointestinal, musculoskeletal, and psychosomatic causes permit work up to be performed at a relatively less expeditious pace.

Angina and Its Mechanism

Angina is a discomfort that follows specific dermatomal pattern being supplied by the spinal cord. The typical features of angina include discomfort in the chest, neck, lower jaw, and radiating towards the arm; whom all are supplied by dermatomes C7-T4 [12]. Thus, angina often radiates to other parts of the body including the upper abdomen, shoulders, arms, fingers, neck, lower jaw, and teeth. Angina follows this distribution pattern irrespective of which area of the myocardium is ischemic. A careful history and physical examination is crucial towards establishing the diagnosis of angina pectoris and to exclude other causes of chest pain.

A thorough assessment of angina based on quality, location and radiation, and associated factors are clinically warranted [13]. Anginal quality is usually difficult to describe. Frequent terms usually described by patients but not limited to include; pressure, tightness, squeezing, constriction, heart burn, elephant sitting on chest, and toothache. The following additional characteristics are typically seen: angina is typically gradual in (may be sudden in case of MI) onset, with the intensity of the discomfort increasing and decreasing over several minutes. Angina is a constant discomfort that does not change with respiration or position. It is also not provoked or worsened with palpation of the chest wall. Patients often indicate the entire chest when asked where the discomfort is felt and to the contrary, pain localized to one small area is generally of pleural or musculoskeletal pain.

Angina is caused by myocardial ischemia, which occurs whenever myocardial oxygen demand exceeds oxygen supply. The mechanisms responsible for angina are complex and not clearly defined. The primary feature of ischemia is decrease in the formation of adenosine triphosphate (ATP), resulting in the development of acidosis, and loss of myocardial membrane function [12]. The release of specific chemical substances such as adenosine, via stimulation of the A1 adenosine receptor that supply innervations to the heart are found to be responsible for angina [14,15]. It is also possible that venodilation plays a role in activate these receptors. Factors that determine myocardial work and myocardial oxygen demand are heart rate, systolic blood pressure, myocardial wall tension, and myocardial contractility. Myocardial contractility and wall tension cannot be measured clinically. As a result, myocardial oxygen demands are estimated clinically by the double product which is a multiplication product of the heart rate and the systolic blood pressure [16].

Symptoms associated with angina are several and the most common is shortness of breath. Other symptoms may include nausea, diaphoresis, dizziness, indigestion, clamminess, and fatigue [17]. However, these symptoms may be seen with other etiologies for chest pain, especially gastrointestinal causes. Chest pain characteristics vary from cardiac to noncardiac causes. Characteristics found to be more typical of nonischemic chest discomfort include, sharp, pleuritic pain related to respiratory movements, pain which is easily reproducible, and constant pain lasting for days or pain lasting for a few seconds(can be included in 3rd paragraph in symptoms along with chest pain characteristics) [18,19]. Special attention needs to be given to patients with diabetes mellitus, who often have autonomic dysfunction and experience silent ischemia However, it is important to remember that some patients with angina present with atypical types of chest pain.

Treatment

Angina is primarily of two type; stable and unstable angina. The primary goals of management for stable angina are relief of symptoms, improvement in quality of life, and survival. This includes three major steps, specifically the modification of coronary artery disease risk factors, pharmacological therapies, and revascularization. All of these steps should be implemented in each patient. For example, all patients should be evaluated for anemia, thyrotoxicosis, tachycardia, and cocaine use as these are conditions that can increase the severity as well as the frequency of angina.

Reduction of coronary risk factors is extremely important. Hypertension plays a crucial role in the management of coronary artery disease. The goal is to decrease blood pressure to less than 140/90, or in the case of diabetes mellitus (DM) or chronic kidney disease (CKD), it should be less 130/80. Dyslipidemia is also a major risk factor in coronary artery disease with reduction of LDL cholesterol to less than 100 mg/dl (or less than 70 mg/dl if patient is a high risk patient) as the primary goal. Lifestyle modifications such as smoking cessation, is one of the most effective steps to prevent progression of atherosclerosis. Evidence also shows that supervised exercise programs can improve tolerance, O2 consumption, and quality of life in conjunction with dietary changes, weight reduction, and control of diabetes mellitus.

Pharmacological therapy consists of a variety of medications including nitrates, beta blockers, calcium channel blockers, and newer anti-anginal agents. Nitrates are a group of medications that cause vascular smooth muscle relaxation and have vasodilator effects on both venous and arterial systems [20]. The mechanism of action involves decreasing both preload and afterload, thereby decreasing oxygen consumption. Nitrates have been shown to improve exercise tolerance and have a synergistic anti-anginal effect when combined with beta blockers or calcium channel blockers. In addition, they can be extremely helpful in vasospastic angina. The most common use of nitrates is sublingually to treat acute episodes of angina. Long acting nitrates such as isosorbide dinitrate and isosorbide mononitrate are used for relief of chronic angina symptoms. Side effects include headache, flushing, and hypotension. Particular caution should be exercised in using continuous administration of nitrates as they are known to cause tachyphylaxis and this can easily be preventable by nitrate-free intervals of at least twelve hours [21]. Nitrates are contraindicated in patients using phosphodiesterase inhibitors or those with right ventricular infarction as it can potentially result in prolonged severe hypotension.

Beta-adrenoceptor blocking agents are used primarily for the reduction in the frequency of anginal episodes as well as increasing the anginal threshold. Beta blockers act by slowing the heart rate, decreasing oxygen consumption, and prolonging diastole which invariably increases coronary perfusion time [22]. Adverse effects include bradycardia, AV blockade, reduced contractility, fatigue, depression, nightmares, bronchoconstriction, GI upset, sexual dysfunction, masking of insulin-induced hypoglycemia, and cutaneous reactions. Beta-1 selective agents should be considered in asthma and COPD patients, however tolerance may be compromised, especially at higher does [23]. Long term therapy with these agents should be slowly withdrawn to avoid precipitation of ischemia in the subsequent several weeks.

Calcium channel blockers inhibit calcium channels in cardiac and vascular smooth muscle membranes. The three major classes are the dihydropyridines (nifedipine, amlodipine and felodipine), the phenylalkylamines (verapamil), and the modified benzodiazepines (diltiazem). The effect is two-fold, decreasing oxygen demand and increasing oxygen supply. Side effects include hypotension, facial flushing, constipation, nausea, headache, dizziness, pedal edema, and rarely gingival hyperplasia. Verapamil acts predominantly as a negative inotrope, amlodipine as a vasodilator, and diltiazem as an intermediary between the two calcium channel blockers.

In addition to nitrates, beta blockers, and calcium channel blockers, a newer agent, ranolazine, was approved by the FDA to treat angina. Ranolazine is a sodium channel blocker that decreases the frequency of angina and increases exercise tolerance[24]. It is typically used as adjunctive therapy when traditional therapy does not provide adequate anginal relief. The main adverse effect is QT prolongation. Nicorandil, Ivabrandine and Fasudil are other anti-anginal agents under investigation.

Along with these medications, aspirin and ACE inhibitors should be used for secondary prevention. Because of mortality benefits, beta blockers are usually the initial agents, unless the patient has severe asthma/COPD, severe symptomatic peripheral vascular disease, or vasospastic angina. In these cases, calcium channel blockers are generally preferred. Moreover, if patient has conduction abnormalities such as sick sinus syndrome or AV nodal disease, amlodipine or nifedipine (not verapamil/diltiazem) can be used. If the patient remains symptomatic while taking beta blockers alone, nitrates or vasodilator calcium channel blockers should be considered as adjunctive therapy. If the patient remains symptomatic despite optimal medical therapy or has high risk features with noninvasive testing, such as a large area of ischemia, patients may benefit from revascularization with balloon angioplasty, stenting, or CABG. Although the burden of evidence did not show improved survival or decreased myocardial infarction with PCI, it did however show improvements in symptoms, exercise tolerance, and quality of life as a whole. CABG is indicated for left main coronary artery disease, triple vessel disease especially with LV dysfunction or diabetes mellitus. Furthermore, revascularization with CABG showed improved survival and better relief of symptoms in comparison to medical therapy.

Conclusion

The term angina is a vague symptom generally described by patients and the mechanisms responsible for the sensation are complex and not clearly defined. Myocardial ischemia occurs whenever myocardial oxygen demand exceeds oxygen supply and evidence points towards adenosine as the primary mediator. Symptomatology of patients with stable angina can be controlled with current medical therapies, such as beta blockers, calcium channel blockers, nitrates, and/or invasive procedures. While some causes of chest pain such as acute myocardial infarction, aortic dissection, or pulmonary embolism require immediate medical intervention, other causes can be worked up in a less time sensitive manner. Coronary artery disease remains the most common etiology of angina with treatment options that are tailored specifically to the three main classifications: stable angina, unstable angina, or acute myocardial infarction.

References

[1]   Lusiani L, Perrone A, Pesavento R, Conte G. Prevalence, clinical features, and acute course of atypical myocardial infarction. *Angiology* 1994; 45:49.

[2]   Longo D, Fauci A, et al. Harrison's Principles of Internal Medicine: Volumes 1 and 2, 18th Edition 2012; 87-98.

[3]   Braunwald E, Zipes DP, et al. Braunwald's Heart Disease: *A Textbook of Cardiovascular Medicine,* 8th Edition.

[4]   Lange RA, Hillis LD. Clinical practice. Acute pericarditis. *N Engl J Med* 2004; 351:2195.

[5]   Phan A, Shufelt C, Merz CN. Persistent chest pain and no obstructive coronary artery disease. *JAMA* 2009; 301:1468.

[6]   Rosen SD, Uren NG, Kaski JC, et al. Coronary vasodilator reserve, pain perception, and sex in patients with syndrome X. *Circulation* 1994; 90:50.

[7]   Kaski JC, Rosano GM, Collins P, et al. Cardiac syndrome X: clinical characteristics and left ventricular function. Long-term follow-up study. *J Am Coll Cardiol* 1995; 25:807.

[8]   Hagan PG, Nienaber CA, Isselbacher EM, et al. The International Registry of Acute Aortic Dissection (IRAD): new insights into an old disease. *JAMA* 2000; 283:897.

[9]   Palla A, Petruzzelli S, Donnamaria V, Giuntini C. The role of suspicion in the diagnosis of pulmonary embolism. *Chest* 1995; 107:21S.

[10]   Stein PD, Beemath A, Matta F, et al. Clinical characteristics of patients with acute pulmonary embolism: data from PIOPED II. *Am J Med* 2007; 120:871.

[11]   Fleet RP, Dupuis G, Marchand A, et al. Panic disorder, chest pain and coronary artery disease: literature review. *Can J Cardiol* 1994; 10:827.

[12]   Foreman RD, Mechanisms of cardiac pain, *Annu Rev Physiol.* 1999;61:143.

[13]   Christie LG Jr, Conti CR, Systematic approach to evaluation of angina-like chest pain: pathophysiology and clinical testing with emphasis on objective documentation of myocardial ischemia. *Am Heart J.* 1981;102(5):897

[14] Gaspardone A, Crea F, Tomai F, Versaci F, Iamele M, GioffrèG, Chiariello L, GioffrèPA, Muscular and cardiac adenosine-induced pain is mediated by A1 receptors. *J Am Coll Cardiol.* 1995;25(1):251.

[15] Crea F, Gaspardone A, Kaski JC, Davies G, Maseri A, Relation between stimulation site of cardiac afferent nerves by adenosine and distribution of cardiac pain: results of a study in patients with stable angina. *J Am Coll Cardiol.* 1992;20(7):1498.

[16] Sonnenblick EH, Ross J, Braunwald E. Oxygen consumption of the heart. Newer concepts of its multifactonal determination. *Am J Cardiol* 1968, 22: 328-36.

[17] Lee TH, Cook EF, Weisberg M, Sargent RK, Wilson C, Goldman L, Acute chest pain in the emergency room. Identification and examination of low-risk patients. *Arch Intern Med.* 1985;145(1):65

[18] Constant J, The clinical diagnosis of nonanginal chest pain: the differentiation of angina from nonanginal chest pain by history. *Clin Cardiol.* 1983;6(1):11.

[19] Panju AA, Hemmelgarn BR, Guyatt GH, Simel DL, The rational clinical examination. Is this patient having a myocardial infarction? *JAMA.* 1998;280(14):1256

[20] Chen Z, Zhang J, Stamler JS. Identification of the enzymatic mechanism of nitroglycerin bioactivation. *Proc Natl Acad Sci U S A.* 2002;99(12):8306.

[21] Parker JD, Parker JO. Nitrate therapy for stable angina pectoris. *N Engl J Med.* 1998;338(8):520.

[22] Gauthier C, Tavernier G, Charpentier F, Langin D, Le Marec H. Functional beta3-adrenoceptor in the human heart. *J Clin Invest.* 1996;98(2):556.

[23] Lertora JJ, Mark AL, Johannsen J, Wilson WR, Abboud FM. Selective beta-1 receptor blockade with oral protocol in man. A dose-related phenomenon. *J Clin Invest.* 1975;56(3):719.

[24] Chaitman BR. Ranolazine for the treatment of chronic angina and potential use in other cardiovascular conditions. *Circulation.* 2006;113(20):2462.

In: Current Issues in the Management of Stable Ischemic Heart ... ISBN: 978-1-62417-203-8
Editor: Mukesh Singh   © 2013 Nova Science Publishers, Inc.

Chapter II

Assessment of Patients with Stable Angina

Jawad M. Khan[*] and Lucy Duckworth
Department of Cardiology, City Hospital, Birmingham, UK

Abstract

This chapter describes the comprehensive assessment of patients with stable angina. The risk factors for coronary artery disease are discussed along with the classification of stable angina symptoms and the initial routine investigations conducted. The array of different invasive and non-invasive diagnostic investigations employed in assessing myocardial ischaemia are presented; exercise electrocardiogram, stress echocardiography, the functional imaging of radionuclide scintigraphy (SPECT), cardiac magnetic resonance imaging (MRI) and multi-detector computed tomography (CT) coronary angiography. The findings of these investigations, including features indicative of high risk and (where applicable) the risk stratification of future cardiac events is discussed along with the tests' sensitivities and specificities. The 'gold standard' investigation of invasive coronary angiography with suitability of patient selection is reviewed. Finally, specific aspects of the investigation of stable angina in diabetic, female and elderly patients are discussed.

Introduction

The assessment of patients who present with chest pain indicative of stable angina should be comprehensive with initial clinical evaluation and routine investigations, followed by diagnostic testing to assess for the presence of myocardial ischaemia. Those individuals who demonstrate low risk features of future cardiac events receive optimal medical therapy with

[*] Address for correspondence: Dr Jawad M Khan, Consultant Interventional Cardiologist and Honorary Senior Clinical Lecturer, Department of Cardiology, City Hospital, Birmingham, UK.

those who show high risk features progressing to coronary angiography with a view to revascularisation. Figure 1 shows the European Society of Cardiology algorithm for the initial evaluation of patients with clinical symptoms of angina [1].

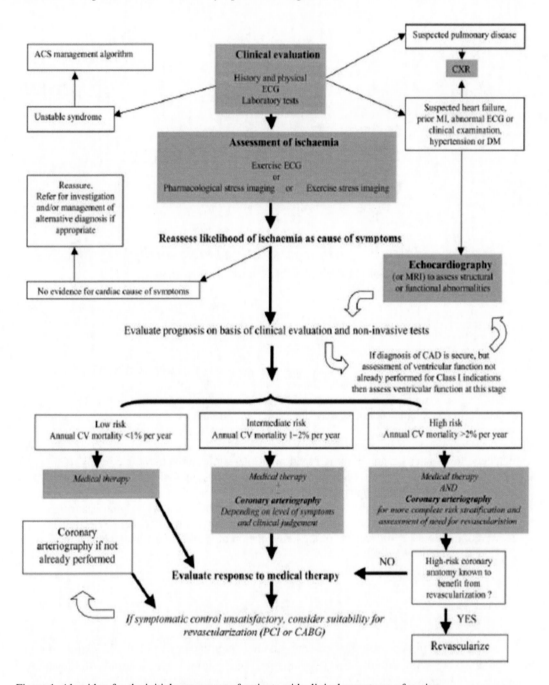

Figure 1. Algorithm for the initial assessment of patients with clinical symptoms of angina.

The method chosen to establish a diagnosis of stable angina following initial assessment is largely dictated by local facilities and expertise. Exercise stress testing is the commonest utilised diagnostic test as it is readily available, relatively cheap to administer and easy to interpret. However, its usefulness is limited by its sensitivity and specificity (68 and 77% respectively) [1].

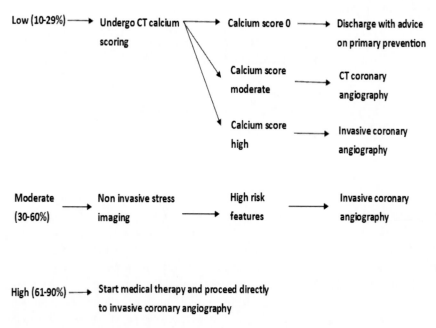

Figure 2. NICE recommended diagnostic investigations based on clinically assessed probability of obstructive coronary artery disease [2].

In March 2010, The UK's National Institute of Health and Clinical Excellence (NICE) published revised guidelines on the assessment of patients presenting with stable cardiac chest pain [2]. They advised that exercise stress electrocardiogram should not be used to diagnose or exclude stable angina, instead, clinical assessment should be undertaken on the likelihood of coronary artery disease based on the patient's age, sex, risk factors and symptoms (Table 1).

Table 1. Percentage of people estimated to have coronary artery disease according to clinical assessment (typicality of symptoms, age, sex and risk factors) [3]

| | Non-anginal chest pain | | | | Atypical angina | | | | Typical angina | | | |
| | Men | | Women | | Men | | Women | | Men | | Women | |
Age (years)	Lo	Hi	Lo	Hi	Lo	Hi	Lo	Hi	Lo	Hi	Lo	Hi
35	3	35	1	19	8	59	2	39	30	88	10	78
45	9	47	2	22	21	70	5	43	51	92	20	79
55	23	59	4	25	45	79	10	47	80	95	38	82
65	49	69	9	29	71	86	20	51	93	97	56	84

For men older than 70 with atypical or typical symptoms, assume an estimate > 90%.
For women older than 70, assume an estimate of 61–90% EXCEPT women at high risk AND with typical symptoms where a risk of > 90% should be assumed.
Hi = High risk = diabetes, smoking and hyperlipidaemia (total cholesterol > 6.47 mmol/litre).
Lo = Low risk = none of these three.

Table 2. Non obstructive coronary disease causes of stable angina

Cardiac
- Hypertrophic Cardiomyopathy
- Aortic Stenosis
- Hypertensive Heart Disease With Left Ventricular Hypertrophy
- Severe Pulmonary Hypertension With Right Ventricular Hypertrophy

Vascular
- Coronary Artery Spasm
- Micro-Vascular Disease (Cardiac Syndrome 'X')

Non Cardiac
- Thyrotoxicosis
- Severe Anaemia

Those patients estimated as being at low probability (10-29%) of significant obstructive coronary disease should undergo computed tomography (CT) calcium scoring, if the calcium score is zero, then patients can be reassured and discharged with advice on primary prevention. If calcium scoring is moderate, then CT coronary angiography is immediately undertaken to demonstrate the presence or absence of coronary artery disease, its location and severity. Individuals who have high calcium scores should progress to coronary angiography. Non-invasive stress imaging is reserved for those individuals who are at moderate probability (30-60%) of having significant obstructive coronary artery, if high risk features are demonstrated on stress imaging then patient's progress to coronary angiography. Patients with high probability of having obstructive coronary artery disease (61-90%) should be commenced on medical therapy for angina and progress directly to coronary angiography [2] (figure 2).

Initial Assessment

Stable angina is caused by an imbalance between the supply and demand for oxygenated blood to the myocardium. The commonest cause is obstructive coronary artery disease. Additional causes of stable angina are shown in table 2. Assessment begins with a careful history and examination to clarify the patient's symptoms, to help identify any non-coronary artery disease causes for angina and to identify risk factors (Table 3).

Symptoms of stable angina are classically described as a pressure sensation or tightness across the chest that may radiate to the arms, jaw and back. They are typically brought on by a predictable level of exertion but can be exacerbated by cold weather and emotional stress or after a heavy meal. Symptoms are usually brief in duration with the sensation of chest discomfort resolving with rest or with the use of sublingual nitrates. Elderly or diabetic patients may present with exertional dyspnoea. The severity of symptoms can be graded by using the Canadian Cardiovascular Society classification (class I to IV) (Table 4).

Table 3. Risk factors for coronary artery disease

- Male sex
- Increasing age
- Smoking
- Increased body mass index (BMI)
- Sedentary life-style
- Diabetes Mellitus
- Hypertension
- Hyperlipidaemia
- South Asian origin

Physical examination may be normal or reveal risk factors for the development of coronary artery disease such as hypertension and obesity. It may also reveal non coronary artery disease causes for angina such as hypertrophic cardiomyopathy, thyrotoxicosis or anaemia. Left ventricular systolic dysfunction as a consequence of ischaemic heart disease may also be identified.

Table 4. The Canadian Cardiovascular Society (CCS) Classification of stable angina

CCS Class	Symptoms
Class I	Angina only occurs with extra-ordinary exertion at work or recreation with ordinary activities not resulting in symptoms.
Class II	Ordinary activity slightly limited by symptoms such as walking more than two blocks on a level surface or climbing more than one flight of stairs at a normal pace.
Class III	Symptoms result in marked limitation of ordinary physical activity such as walking one to two blocks on a level surface or climbing one flight of stairs at normal pace.
Class IV	Chest discomfort occurs at minimal activity or stress or at rest.

Table 5. Features that indicate higher risk of future cardiac events

- Early positive test (less than 3 minutes of the standard Bruce protocol).
- A strongly positive test (more than 2 mm ST segment depression); with sustained ST segment depression after exercise cessation (more than 3 minutes).
- Ischaemia at low heart rate (less than 120 beats per minute).
- Blunted blood pressure response to exercise or a reduction in blood pressure at peak exercise.
- Significant ventricular arrhythmias at low workload (less than 120 beats per minute).
- Inability to complete two stages of the standard Bruce protocol (i.e. less than 6 minutes of exercise).

Initial Investigations

Initial investigations include full blood count, renal function, fasting blood glucose, fasting lipid profile (total cholesterol, low density lipoprotein (LDL) cholesterol, high density lipoprotein (HDL) cholesterol and triglycerides) and thyroid function tests.

A baseline electrocardiogram (ECG) should also be undertaken. A normal ECG does not exclude the presence of coronary artery disease although the presence of ST segment depression or T wave inversion may be indicative of the presence of ischaemic heart disease and the presence of Q waves or left bundle branch block would indicate previous myocardial injury and are associated with unfavourable outcome. Left ventricular hypertrophy is suggested by increased QRS complex size and can occur in hypertension but may also be a finding in the context of severe aortic stenosis.

Echocardiography may show regional wall motion abnormalities with areas of hypokinesia (reduced wall motion and thickening during contraction) indicating the presence of coronary artery disease. Echocardiography may also identify non coronary causes of angina such as hypertrophic cardiomyopathy and severe aortic stenosis. As left ventricular systolic function declines, mortality increases. A resting ejection fraction of less than 35% is associated with a greater than 3% annual mortality rate [4-7].

Although a chest x-ray does not provide specific information for the diagnosis or risk stratification of stable angina, it should be undertaken in patients with suspected heart failure, valvular or pulmonary disease. The presence of pulmonary congestion, cardiomegaly, atrial enlargement and cardiac calcification have been related to adverse prognosis [5, 8].

Ambulatory ECG monitoring has a role in patients with vasospastic angina or to detect silent ischemia. It is also useful when tachy-arrhythmias are suspected as a cause of the patients symptoms. A sudden increase in the patient's heart rate secondary to an arrhythmia may explain the occurrence of episodic angina at rest.

Non Invasive Cardiac Investigations

Non-invasive methods of assessing myocardial ischaemia involve applying a stress to the myocardium in order to provoke myocardial ischaemia or to produce coronary artery vasodilatation. The stress is then followed by a method of assessing the resultant ischaemia or differential perfusion.

The most useful and physiological method of inducing myocardial ischaemia is through exercise. For those individuals who are unable to exercise, pharmacological methods can be utilised. An exercise test is considered adequate if the patient achieves more than 85% of their maximum age predicted heart rate per minute (220 minus the patient's age) [9].

Pharmacological methods include dobutamine, adenosine and dipyridamole. Dobutamine is a beta 1 receptor agonist and at low doses has a positive inotropic effect resulting in increased force of contraction of the left ventricle. At higher doses, it produces an additional increase in heart rate (chronotropic effect). The plasma half-life of dobutamine is 2 to 3 minutes. An incremental dobutamine infusion produces similar effects to exercise and adequate stress is defined as a heart rate that increases to more than 85% of the maximum age predicted heart rate. If, despite high doses of dobutamine, the heart rate remains below this level then intravenous atropine can be given.

Adenosine causes coronary micro-vascular vasodilatation and results in a discrepancy in myocardial blood flow with increased perfusion to areas of the myocardium supplied by normal arteries, with areas of the myocardium supplied by stenosed vessels unable to increase blood flow. Perfusion in this area may also be reduced by coronary steal with blood preferentially being diverted to areas of micro-vascular vasodilatation.

Dipyridamole also causes coronary micro-vascular vasodilatation but does so by inhibiting the cellular uptake of adenosine. This onset of action is slower but is of longer duration. It is important to ensure that patients are not already on dipyridamole for other reasons (e.g. cerebrovascular disease). Caffeine should be avoided for 12 to 24 hours prior to the study, as it interferes with the metabolism of dipyridamole. Adenosine should be avoided in asthmatics as it can induce bronchospasm.

In general, pharmacological stress is safe and well tolerated by patients. Major cardiac complications, including sustained ventricular tachycardia, occurs in one out of 1500 stress tests with dipyridamole or adenosine and 1 in every 300 stress tests with dobutamine [10].

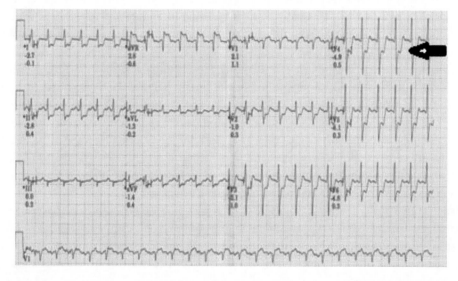

Figure 3. A 12 lead ECG showing widespread marked horizontal ST segment depression during stage II of the Standard Bruce Protocol at a heart rate of 148/min, 93% of the patients max age predicted heart rate (220 minus age 60 years).

Methods of Assessing Myocardial Ischaemia

12 Lead Electrocardiogram (ECG)

A continuously recorded 12 lead ECG during the application of stress can be indicative of the presence of myocardial ischaemia demonstrated by the development of horizontal ST segment depression with the onset of typical symptoms. A test can be considered positive if the patient develops 1 mm ST segment depression (0.1 mv for ≥ 60 to 80 milliseconds after the end of the QRS complex), in the context of the development of chest pain (Figure 3).

The reported sensitivity and specificity for the detection of coronary artery disease with exercise stress ECG is 70 and 77% respectively [11, 12]. Increasing the threshold for a positive test to ≥2mm (0.2 mV) ST segment depression will increase specificity at the expense of sensitivity. Various exercise protocols exist with the most popular being the standard Bruce protocol, involving 3 minute stages of increasing exercise resulting from altering the speed and gradient of a treadmill. Protocols involving leg or upper arm cycle machines also exist. In addition to heart rate, workload can also be expressed as oxygen uptake in multiples of resting requirements. One metabolic equivalent (MET) is a unit of sitting or resting oxygen uptake (3.5 ml of oxygen per kg body weight per minute) [13].

In the CASS Registry [7], 12% of medically treated patients were identified as high risk on the basis of ≥1mm exercise induced ST-segment depression and inability to complete stage I of the Standard Bruce Protocol. These individuals had an average mortality of 5 % per year. Of the patients, 34% could exercise to Stage III of the standard Bruce protocol without ST segment changes; they were defined as low risk and had an annual mortality of less than 1%. [7].

A patient's risk can also be calculated by the Duke Treadmill Score (DTS) [14]. This is a validated scoring system that combines exercise time, ST segment deviation and the occurrence of angina. The DTS equals the exercise time in minutes minus (five times the ST segment deviation in millimetres, during exercise or in recovery) minus (four times the angina index).

The angina index is 0 if the patient experienced no angina during the test, 1 if angina occurred and 2 if the test was stopped due to the angina (figure 4). Two thirds of patients whose score indicated low risk had a four year survival rate of 99% (i.e. average annual mortality rate of 0.25%), whereas 4% had a DTS indicating high risk, their four year survival was 79% (average annual mortality of 5%) [14]. In addition to clinical assessment, the DTS provides an effective method of discriminating between low and high risk patients [14].

Patients that demonstrate features on exercise stress testing indicating high risk of future cardiac events should progress to coronary angiography (Table 5).

False positive tests are more frequent in the presence of left ventricular hypertrophy. Myocardial ischaemia cannot be excluded in the context of a sub maximal test (i.e. an achieved heart rate less than 85% of the maximum age predicted heart rate). Also, a normal test in patients taking anti-ischaemic medication does not exclude the presence of significant coronary artery disease [15].

Therefore, for diagnostic exercise stress ECG tests anti-ischaemic drugs should be stopped for 48 hours prior to the test. However, this may not always be possible or safe to do so.

When exercise ECG testing is used for the assessment of significant coronary disease in women, there is a high false positive rate (38-67%) compared to men (7-44%) [16]. This is mainly due to the lower pre-test probability of disease [17] but also a lower false-negative rate in women [18].

For this reason, stress imaging is the preferred diagnostic modality in women. However, the sensitivity of radionuclide perfusion imaging is lower in women compared to men [19]. Breast attenuation artifact may result in an apparent anterior perfusion defects, this can be reduced by using gated imaging [20]

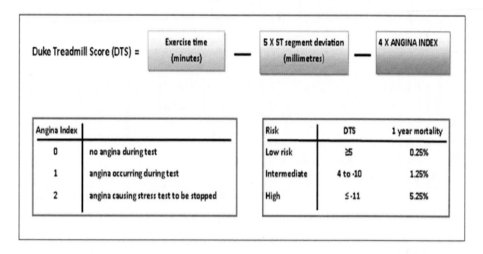

Figure 4. Duke Treadmill Score.

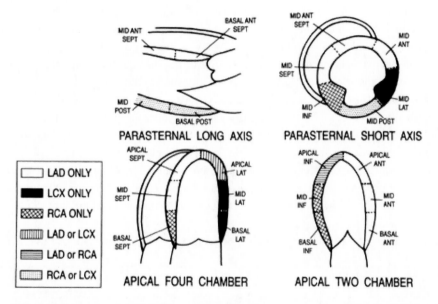

Figure 5. 16-segment model showing segments supplied by the major epicardial vessels. LAD indicates left anterior descending coronary artery; LCX, left circumflex coronary artery; RCA, right coronary artery; MID, mid ventricular; ANT, anterior; SEPT, septal; POST, posterior; LAT, lateral; INF, inferior.

Complications during exercise testing are uncommon but severe arrhythmias, ST segment elevation myocardial infarction or even sudden cardiac death can occur. The rate of death and myocardial infarction is less than 1 in 2500 tests [21]. Table 6 lists contra-indications to exercise testing and these should be checked by the referring physician. A physician should be present or immediately available to monitor the test and the cardiac physiologists who conducts the test should be trained to administer immediate life support (ILS). A defibrillator should also be available to manage ischaemia induced pulseless ventricular tachycardia or ventricular fibrillation.

Table 6. The contra-indications to diagnostic exercise stress testing

- Uncontrolled hypertension (>200 mmHg systolic and/or >110 mmHg diastolic)
- Left bundle branch block on the baseline ECG or a paced rhythm
- Suspected unstable angina or acute myocardial infarction
- Acute myocarditis or pericarditis
- Symptomatic severe aortic stenosis
- Uncontrolled, symptomatic heart failure
- Uncontrolled arrhythmia
- Inability to perform an exercise ECG due to co-morbidity or disability

Echocardiography

Echocardiography, undertaken continuously during the application of stress (cycle exercise machine or dobutamine infusion) allows an assessment of reversible myocardial ischaemia, viability and the presence of scar. Areas of the myocardium supplied by stenosed vessels exhibit normal wall motion and thickening at rest but become hypokinetic (less than 50% normal wall motion) with stress. Scar tissue shows a resting abnormality (usually akinesia- no contraction or thickening of that myocardial segment) which does not improve with the application of stress. Hibernating myocardium shows hypokinesia or akinesia at rest but with the application of stress, wall motion improves only to deteriorate again once the myocardium becomes more ischaemic (Table 7). Stress echocardiogram can effectively risk stratify patients and has excellent negative predictive value [22]. The reported sensitivity and specificity of dobutamine stress echo ranges from 40 to 100% and 62 to 100% respectively [10]. Beta blockers should be stopped for 48 hours prior to the stress test if safe to do so.

Table 7. The interpretation of wall motion abnormalities in response to stress

Interpretation	Baseline	Low Level Stress	Peak and Post Stress Function
Normal	Normal	Normal or Hyper-dynamic Response	Hyper-dynamic response
Ischaemia	Normal	Normal or in the context of severe coronary artery disease can deteriorate	Deterioration (development of hypokinesia or akinesia)
Viable and Ischaemic (hibernating)	Resting regional wall abnormality	Improved motion	Deterioration (development of hypokinesia or akinesia)
Scar Tissue	Resting regional wall abnormality (usually akinetic)	No change	No change

Stress echocardiography [23] allows risk stratification for future cardiac events. Although the occurrence of regional wall motion abnormality with stress indicates the presence of coronary artery disease, the severity or extent of coronary artery disease relates to the number of segments that become hypokinetic and the level of stress that is required to induce myocardial ischaemia and hence regional wall motion abnormality (heart rate and dose of dobutamine) (Table 8). The regional abnormality can help predict the epicardial coronary vessel responsible (Figure 5).

Stress echocardiography is limited by the quality of echo images and, in approximately 33% of patients [24]; the image quality is sufficiently sub-optimal to preclude the test. Improvements in technology include enhanced endocardial border definition with the use of intravenous contrast media which facilitates identification of regional wall motion abnormalities [25].

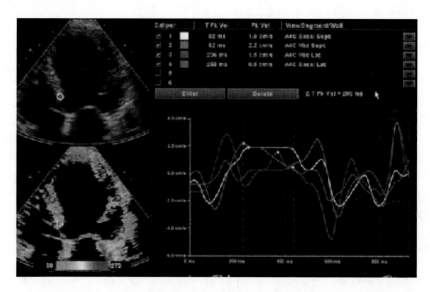

Figure 6. Tissue doppler imaging allowing accurate assessment of wall motion and velocity.

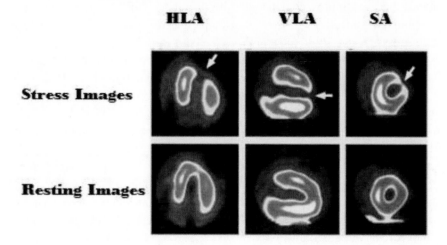

Figure 7. Shows a reversible perfusion defect at the apex and anterior wall (arrows). (HLA, horizontal long axis; VLA, vertical long axis; SA, short axis).

Table 8. Risk stratification with stress echocardiography

Finding on stress echocardiography	Degree of risk
Extensive ischaemia with wall motion abnormality involving >2 segments developing at low dose of dobutamine (<10mcg/kg/min) or at a low heart rate (<120 beats/min)	High (annual cardiovascular mortality of >3%)
• Mild/moderate resting LV dysfunction (LVEF 35% - 49%) • Limited ischaemia with a wall motion abnormality involving < 2 segments only at higher doses of dobutamine	Moderate (annual cardiovascular mortality of 1-3%)
• Normal wall motion or no change of limited resting wall motion abnormalities during stress	Low (annual cardiovascular mortality of <1%)

The use of tissue doppler imaging (figure 6) allows quantification of regional wall motion abnormalities (velocity). Strain and strain rate imaging allow regional deformation to be determined. Strain relates to the difference in the velocity of adjacent regions of the myocardium with the strain rate being difference per unit length. These techniques have improved the diagnostic ability of dobutamine stress echo to detect ischemia and provide a more objective assessment method [26].

Radionuclide Scintigraphy (SPECT)

This imaging modality involves single photon emission computed tomography (SPECT) which utilises radio-pharmaceuticals such as thallium 201 and technetium 99^{m}. With thallium, relative myocardial ischemia is demonstrated by differences in the distribution of thallium. With technetium, two injections of the radioisotope are given comparing the uptake during rest and with stress.

Reversible defects between stress and rest indicate reversible myocardial ischemia (Figure 7) with fixed defects indicating previous myocardial infarction. Patients who are found to have abnormal perfusion defects are at 15 fold higher risk of mortality from cardiovascular causes compared to those individuals who have normal scans [24]. The greatest risk is associated with those scans showing multiple segments of abnormal perfusion or large defects especially involving the anterior wall.

The proximal septum correlates to proximal left anterior descending artery stenosis and reversible ischemia in this segment also indicates poor prognosis. Demonstration of lung uptake and exercise induced dilatation of the left ventricle are markers of severe coronary artery disease [24, 27]. High risk features on myocardial perfusion imaging should prompt progression to coronary angiography.

A normal stress perfusion study is associated with a cardiac death and myocardial infarction rate of less than 1% per year which is equivalent to that of the general population. [28].

The sensitivity and specificity for the detection of coronary artery disease with adenosine stress SPECT ranges from 83 to 94% and 64 to 90% respectively [29]. Stress imaging should not be undertaken if contra-indications exist and these should be assessed by the referring physician (Table 9).

Table 9. Contra indications to stress imaging include

- Uncontrolled hypertension (more than 200 mmHg systolic and or more than 110 mmHg diastolic)
- Suspected unstable angina or acute myocardial infarction.
- Acute myocarditis or pericarditis
- Uncontrolled, symptomatic heart failure
- Symptomatic severe aortic stenosis.

Table 10. A summary of test characteristics for investigations used in the diagnosis of stable angina [1]

	Diagnosis of CAD	
	Sensitivity (%)	Specificity (%)
Exercise ECG	68	77
Exercise echo	80-85	84-86
Exercise myocardial perfusion	85-90	70-75
Dobutamine stress echo	40-100	62-100
Vasodilator stress echo	56-92	87-100
Vasodilator stress myocardial perfusion	83-94	64-90

Stress Cardiac Magnetic Resonance (CMR)

CMR stress testing, with dobutamine infusion as the stress, can be used to detect regional wall motion abnormalities as a result of myocardial ischaemia.

Due to the high quality images, this technique has been shown to compare favourably to dobutamine stress echo [30]. Additionally, delay in first pass gadolinium allows an assessment of myocardial perfusion (Figure 8) with late gadolinium enhancement identifying infarcted tissue (Figure 9). The use of stress CMR is limited primarily due to limited availability.

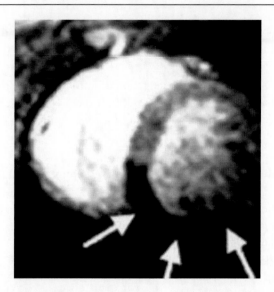

Figure 8. Cardiac MRI of the right and left ventricle with delayed first pass gadolinium (arrows) indicating reduced perfusion to the inferior and infero-septal walls of the left ventricle consistent with a right coronary artery stenosis.

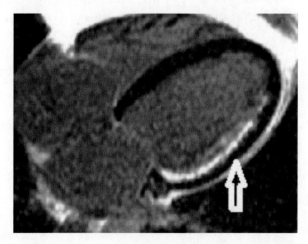

Figure 9. Cardiac MRI of the left ventricle with late hyper-enhancement with gadolinium of the lateral wall (arrow) indicating infarcted scar tissue in the sub-endocardial region due to previous non ST elevation myocardial infarction with a plaque rupture event in the circumflex coronary artery.

Multi Detector Coronary Computed Tomography

The use of CT to image the heart was previously limited by spatial resolution and movement artifact. However the development of multi detector CT enhanced by ECG gating and the use of intravenous contrast media have advanced this technique and have allowed sensitivities and specificities of over 89% and 96% respectively with a 98% negative predictive value [31]. Calcium scoring can be used as an indirect assessment of the severity of coronary artery disease. Calcium is deposited in atherosclerotic plaques within the coronary arteries. The level of calcification increases with age and established nomograms exist giving expected values for calcium scores with respect to age and gender. The Agatston score [32] is a commonly used scoring system for calcium and is based on the density and area of calcified plaques, providing an assessment of the risk of significant coronary artery disease. Those individuals with moderate calcium scores proceed directly to CT coronary angiography (figure 10) and high calcium scores, to invasive coronary angiography [2]. The main limitation with CT coronary angiography is that it provides good anatomical data but no functional data as to the significance of any coronary artery stenosis identified. Newer hybrid machines combine CT with a gamma camera which allows SPECT scanning with functional assessment in the form of perfusion defects that can then be correlated with any coronary artery stenosis identified on CT coronary angiography.

Coronary Angiography

The gold standard for accurate detection of coronary artery stenosis remains coronary angiography (Figure 11). Although this is an invasive test, the risk of coronary angiography (1 in 1000 risk of myocardial infarction, stroke and death) [33] is justified in those individuals estimated to be at high risk of future cardiac events and likely to require revascularisation. Functional significance of individual lesions identified on coronary angiography can be determined further with pressure wire assessment (fractional flow reserve). The use of intravascular ultrasound provides additional information with regards to lesion morphology, plaque burden and severity and allows optimisation of stent deployment.

Coronary angiography is recommended for those patients with [1]:

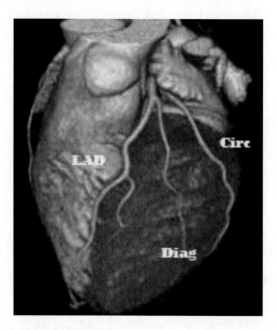

Figure 10. CT coronary angiography identifying the left coronary circulation (LAD, left anterior descending artery; Circ, circumflex artery; Diag, diagonal artery).

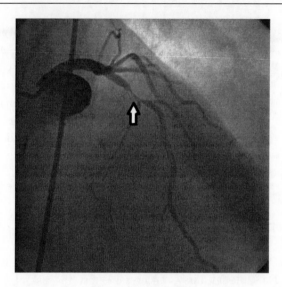

Figure 11. Shows a severe (>70%) stenosis in the mid left anterior descending artery on invasive coronary angiography.

1 Inadequate control of symptoms despite optimal medical therapy.
2 Those patients who have high risk features on stress testing.
3 Patients with moderate to severely impaired left ventricular systolic function.
4 Those requiring major surgical intervention.
5 Patients previously treated with myocardial revascularisation (PCI or coronary artery bypass graft surgery) who then develop early recurrence with limiting angina.
6 Patients with serious ventricular arrhythmias.
7 Patients who survive cardiac arrest.
8 Patients with inconclusive diagnosis on non-invasive testing.

Demonstration of coronary artery disease is associated with an increased risk of future cardiac events. A coronary artery stenosis greater than 70% is sufficient to result in flow limitation with resultant myocardial ischemia. However, the severity of a particular stenosis does not predict plaque stability. The majority of patients who develop acute myocardial infarction, due to coronary artery occlusion, have a 50% or less diameter stenosis at the site of occurrence of plaque rupture resulting in the myocardial infarction [34, 35].

Management in Special Groups

Diabetic Patients

The cardiac assessment of symptomatic diabetic patients, in general, should mirror that of non-diabetics with similar indications for exercise testing, myocardial perfusion imaging and coronary angiography. However, with the use of 24 hour ambulatory ECG, it is estimated that up to two thirds of myocardial ischaemic episodes are silent [36-38]. In asymptomatic men between 40-59 years, the prevalence of silent ischaemia as determined by coronary angiography is 0.89% [39] with other studies suggesting 1-4% prevalence [40, 41]. This rises in asymptomatic diabetic individuals to 10-20% [42, 43], thus adding to the complexity of managing coronary artery disease in diabetic patients. In the MRFIT trial [44], there was a significant relationship between silent ischaemia and mortality in asymptomatic diabetic and non-diabetic men due to silent ischaemia confirming the presence of significant coronary disease. Also, repeated ischaemic episodes results in progressive myocardial fibrosis, progression to left ventricular dysfunction and malignant arrhythmias.

Routine screening of all asymptomatic diabetic patients is currently not recommended. However, asymptomatic diabetic patients who have two or more risk factors for the development of coronary artery disease, or predictive clinical markers, should be screened for silent ischaemia with an exercise tolerance test (ETT) [45]. An alternative would be CT calcium scoring (depending on the facilities and expertise available). If the ETT is negative, or normal CT calcium score, then patients should be reassured that at this point in time they are unlikely to have significant obstructive coronary disease; with the priority being to achieve good glycaemic control and modify risk factors. Patients with moderate calcium scores should proceed to CT coronary angiography. If the ETT is equivocal, patients have limited mobility or impaired left ventricular function; myocardial perfusion imaging or dobutamine stress echocardiography should be undertaken for clarification. Those individuals with a positive ETT or high calcium score should proceed to invasive coronary angiography.

Conventional Risk Factors

Smoking, hypertension, hypercholesterolemia, family history and micro-albuminuria are risk factors for the development of atherosclerotic vascular disease in diabetic patients. In the DIAD study [46], diabetic patients with two or more risk factors were more likely to have prognostically significant disease and should, therefore, undergo screening for the presence of silent myocardial ischaemia, if asymptomatic, with conventional stress testing.

Predictive Clinical Markers

Predictive clinical markers for coronary artery disease in diabetes include breathlessness, abnormal resting ECG, peripheral vascular disease, cardiac autonomic neuropathy and erectile dysfunction [46].

Breathlessness on Exertion

This may signify silent myocardial ischaemia or 'angina equivalent'. Diabetic patients with breathlessness are significantly more likely to have myocardial ischaemia with a worse outcome compared to those diabetics who are completely asymptomatic or who are symptomatic with angina [47]. Breathlessness may also represent impaired left ventricular function which is associated with adverse outcome. However, breathlessness in diabetics is often multifactorial and may reflect increased body mass index, hypertension with diastolic dysfunction and respiratory disease, making assessment difficult.

Abnormal Resting ECG

Non-specific ST and T wave changes on the resting ECG are strong predictors of silent ischaemia. Additionally, 43% of diabetics with Q waves and 26% with ST-T wave changes had high risk features on subsequent myocardial perfusion imaging (MPI) [47]. The majority of those with high risk features on MPI having prognostically significant coronary artery disease [48].

Peripheral Vascular Disease (PVD)

High risk MPI results were found in 28% of patients with peripheral vascular disease (PVD), with 47% of asymptomatic diabetics with PVD demonstrating silent ischaemia and 37% with evidence of prior silent myocardial infarction [49,50].

Cardiac Autonomic Neuropathy (CAN)

In diabetic patients, CAN is suggested by a postural reduction in blood pressure, reduced heart rate variability or unexplained resting tachycardia. CAN is associated with an increased prevalence of silent myocardial ischaemia (64.7% compared to 4.1% in non-diabetics), myocardial infarction and poor prognosis in diabetics [51, 52].

Erectile Dysfunction (ED)

ED doubles the incidence of future coronary artery disease (CAD) in diabetic patients without known CAD [53]. There was a 33.8% prevalence of ED in diabetics with silent CAD compared to 4.7% in those without silent ischaemia [54]. ED was a better predictor of silent CAD that smoking, micro-albuminuria and LDL- cholesterol concentration [48].

Female Patients

Stable angina is the most frequent first manifestation of CAD in women, with men presenting mainly with myocardial infarction or sudden cardiac death [55-57]. In the post-menopausal age group, the incidence of angina in women exceeds that in men. The majority of women present with typical symptoms of angina, although an atypical presentation is more common than in men, with differences in female patient perception of pain and terminology used [58]. Cardiac syndrome X is also more common in women as is coronary vasospasm.

When exercise ECG testing is used for the assessment of significant coronary disease in women, there is a high false positive rate (38-67%) compared to men (7-44%) [16]. This is mainly due to the lower pre-test probability of disease [17] but also a lower false-negative rate in women [18]. For this reason, stress imaging is the preferred diagnostic modality in women. However, the sensitivity of radionuclide perfusion imaging is lower in women compared to men [19]. Breast attenuation artifact may manifest in anterior perfusion defects, this can be reduced by using gated imaging [20]. NICE guidance has recommended the use of CT calcium scoring in men and women at low risk (on clinical assessment) of having obstructive coronary disease [2]. The Euro Heart Survey of stable angina showed a significant bias against the use of coronary angiography and exercise testing in women compared to men, they were also less likely to proceed to revascularisation [53].

Elderly Patients

The prevalence of CAD is similar in men and women after the age of 75 years. These patients are more likely to have severe and diffuse CAD (three vessel disease and left main artery stenosis) and impaired left ventricular systolic function. Reduced activity levels and less appreciation of ischaemic symptoms are more common with advancing age [60] with muscle weakness, joint disease and deconditioning contributing to the reduction in functional capacity. Hypertension with diastolic impairment, valvular heart disease and conduction abnormalities are also more common with increasing age. This limits the usefulness of exercise stress testing. ETT is also associated with increased risk of ischaemia related arrhythmias [61]. Pharmacological stress testing should be employed in elderly patients who are deemed to be unsuitable for exercise testing. NICE guidance [2] directs towards the use of coronary angiography in symptomatic elderly patients. It is important to note that elective diagnostic coronary angiography has relatively little increased risk compared to younger patients [62] although the incidence of contrast induced nephropathy is increased in patients over the age of 75 years [63].

Conclusion

The assessment of patients who present with chest pain indicative of stable angina should be comprehensive with initial clinical evaluation and routine investigations, followed by diagnostic testing to assess for the presence of myocardial ischaemia. The method chosen to establish a diagnosis of stable angina following initial assessment is largely dictated by local facilities and expertise. There is a move away from non-invasive testing with relatively low sensitivity and specificity (exercise stress ECG) with adoption of new imaging modalities (CT calcium scoring and coronary angiography with combined SPECT). Those individuals who demonstrate low risk features of future cardiac events, on non-invasive testing, receive optimal medical therapy with those who show high risk features progressing to coronary angiography with a view to revascularisation. At initial assessment, if the probability of having significant coronary artery disease is high then, to minimise delay to diagnosis, patients should start medical therapy and move directly to invasive coronary angiography with a view to revascularisation, if indicated.

References

[1] Kim Fox, Maria Angeles Alonso Garcia, Diego Ardissino, Pawel Buszma, Poala G Camici, Filippo Crea, Caroline Daly, Guy De Becker, Paul Hjemdahl, Jose Lopez-Sendon, Jean Marco, Joao Moruis, John Pepper, Ado Sechtem, Maarten Simons, Kristan Thygesen. Guidelines on the management of angina pectoris. *European Heart Journal* 2006; 27:1341-1381.

[2] www.nice.org.uk/guidance/CG95

[3] Adapted from Pryor DB, Shaw L, McCants CB et al. (1993) Value of the history and physical in identifying patients at increased risk for coronary artery disease. *Annals of Internal Medicine* 118(2): 81–90.

[4] Mock MB, Ringqvist I, Fisher LD, Davis KB, Chaitman BR, Kouchoukos NT et al. Survival of medically treated patients in the coronary artery surgery study (CASS) registry. *Circulation* 1982;66:562–568.

[5] Weiner DA, Ryan TJ, McCabe CH, Chaitman BR, Sheffield LT, Ferguson JC et al. Prognostic importance of a clinical profile and exercise test in medically treated patients with coronary artery disease. *J Am Coll Cardiol* 1984;3:772–779.

[6] Hammermeister KE, DeRouen TA, Dodge HT. Variables predictive of survival in patients with coronary disease. Selection by univariate and multivariate analyses from the clinical, electrocardiographic, exercise, arteriographic, and quantitative angiographic evaluations. *Circulation* 1979;59:421–430.

[7] Emond M, Mock MB, Davis KB, Fisher LD, Holmes DR Jr, Chaitman BR et al. Long-term survival of medically treated patients in the Coronary Artery Surgery Study (CASS) Registry. *Circulation* 1994;90:2645–2657.

[8] Hemingway H, Shipley M, Christie D, Marmot M. Cardiothoracic ratio and relative heart volume as predictors of coronary heart disease mortality. The Whitehall study 25 year follow-up. *Eur Heart J* 1998;19:859–869.

[9] Fox III SM, Naughton JP and Haskell WL. Physical activity and the prevention of coronary heart disease. *Ann Clin Res* 1971; 3:404-432.

[10] Marwick TH. Current status of stress echocardiography for diagnosis and prognostic assessment of coronary artery disease. *Coron Artery Dis.* 1998;9:411–426.

[11] Gianrossi R, Detrano R, Mulvihill D, Lehmann K, Dubach P, Colombo A et al. Exercise-induced ST depression in the diagnosis of coronary artery disease. A meta-analysis. *Circulation* 1989; 80:87–98.

[12] Ashley EA, Myers J, Froelicher V. Exercise testing in clinical medicine. *Lancet* 2000; 356:1592–1597.

[13] Jette M, Sidney K, Blumchen G. Metabolic equivalents (METS) in exercise testing, exercise prescription, and evaluation of functional capacity. *Clin Cardiol* 1990;13:555–565.

[14] Mark DB, Shaw L, Harrell FE Jr, Hlatky MA, Lee KL, Bengtson JR et al. Prognostic value of a treadmill exercise score in outpatients with suspected coronary artery disease. *N Engl J Med* 1991;325:849–853.

[15] ESC Working Group on Exercise Physiology, Physiopathology and Electro-cardiography. Guidelines for cardiac exercise testing. *Eur Heart J* 1993;14:969–988.

[16] Gibbons RJ, Balady GJ, Bricker JT, Chaitman BR, Fletcher GF, Froelicher VF et al. ACC/AHA 2002 guideline update for exercise testing: summary article. A report of the American College of Cardiology/American Heart Association Task Force on Practice Guidelines (Committee to Update the 1997 Exercise Testing Guidelines). *J Am Coll Cardiol* 2002;40:1531–1540

[17] Diamond GA, Forrester JS. Analysis of probability as an aid in the clinical diagnosis of coronary-artery disease. *N Engl J Med* 1979;300:1350–1358.

[18] Villareal RPWJ. Noninvasive diagnostic testing. In: Wilansky SWJ, ed. *Heart Disease in Women.* Philadelphia: Churchill Livingstone; 2002. P149–157.

[19] Osbakken MD, Okada RD, Boucher CA et al. Comparison of exercise perfusion and ventricular function imaging: an analysis of factors affecting the diagnostic accuracy of each technique. *J Am Coll Cardiol* 1984;3:272–283.

[20] DePuey EG, Rozanski A. Using gated technetium-99m-sestamibi SPECT to characterize fixed myocardial defects as infarct or artifact. *J Nucl Med* 1995;36:952–955.

[21] Stuart RJ Jr, Ellestad MH. National survey of exercise stress testing facilities. *Chest* 1980;77:94–97.

[22] Geleijnse ML, Elhendy A, van Domburg RT, Cornel JH, Rambaldi R, Salustri A et al. Cardiac imaging for risk stratification with dobutamine-atropine stress testing in patients with chest pain. Echocardiography, perfusion scintigraphy, or both? *Circulation* 1997;96:137–147.

[23] Schinkel AF, Bax JJ, Geleijnse ML, Boersma E, Elhendy A, Roelandt JR et al. Noninvasive evaluation of ischaemic heart disease: myocardial perfusion imaging or stress echocardiography? *Eur Heart J* 2003;24:789–800.

[24] Korosoglou G, Labadze N, Hansen A, Selter C, Giannitsis E, Katus H et al. Usefulness of real-time myocardial perfusion imaging in the evaluation of patients with first time chest pain. *Am J Cardiol* 2004; 94:1225–1231.

[25] Thanigaraj S, Nease RF, Schechtman KB et al. Use of contrast for image enhancement during stress echocardiography is cost-effective and reduces additional diagnostic testing. *Am J Cardiol* 2001; 87:1430–2.

[26] Madler CF, Payne N, Wilkenshoff U, Cohen A, Derumeaux GA, Pierard LA et al. Non-invasive diagnosis of coronary artery disease by quantitative stress echocardiography: optimal diagnostic models using off-line tissue doppler in the MYDISE study. *Eur Heart J* 2003; 24:1584–1594.

[27] Underwood SR, Anagnostopoulos C, Cerqueira M, Ell PJ, Flint EJ, Harbinson M et al. Myocardial perfusion scintigraphy: the evidence. *Eur J Nucl Med Mol Imaging* 2004; 31:261–291.

[28] Zaret BL, Wackers FJ. Nuclear cardiology (1). *N Engl J Med* 1993;329: 775–783.

[29] Gibbons RJ, Chatterjee K, Daley J, Douglas JS, Fihn SD, Gardin JM et al. ACC/AHA/ACP-ASIM guidelines for the management of patients with chronic stable angina: a report of the American College of Cardiology/American Heart Association Task Force on Practice Guidelines (Committee on Management of Patients With Chronic Stable Angina). *J Am Coll Cardiol* 1999; 33:2092–2197.

[30] Hundley WG, Hamilton CA, Clarke GD, Hillis LD, Herrington DM, Lange RA et al. Visualization and functional assessment of proximal and middle left anterior

descending coronary stenoses in humans with magnetic resonance imaging. *Circulation* 1999; 99:3248–3254.

[31] Schroeder S, Achenbach S, Bengel F, et al. Cardiac computed tomography: indications, applications, limitations, and training requirements: report of a Writing Group deployed by the Working Group Nuclear Cardiology and Cardiac CT of the European Society of Cardiology and the European Council of Nuclear Cardiology. *Eur Heart J* 2008; 29:531-56.

[32] Agatston AS, Janowitz WR, Hildner FJ, Zusmer NR, Viamonte M Jr, Detrano R. Quantification of coronary artery calcium using ultrafast computed tomography. *J Am Coll Cardiol* 1990; 15:827–832.

[33] Noto TJ Jr, Johnson LW, Krone R, et al. Cardiac catheterization 1990: a report of the Registry of the Society for Cardiac Angiography and Interventions (SCAandI). *Cathet Cardiovasc Diagn.* 1991;24:75–83

[34] Ambrose JA, Winters SL, Arora RR, et al. Coronary angiographic morphology in myocardial infarction: a link between the pathogenesis of unstable angina and myocardial infarction. *J Am Coll Cardiol.* 1985; 6:1233–1238.

[35] Ambrose JA, Tannenbaum MA, Alexopoulos D, et al. Angiographic progression of coronary artery disease and the development of myocardial infarction. *J Am Coll Cardiol.* 1988;12:56–62.

[36] Deedwania PC, Carbajal EV. Silent myocardial ischemia: a clinical perspective. *Arch Intern Med* 1991; 151:2373-82.

[37] L angou RA, Huang EK, Kelley MK et al. Predictive accuracy of coronary artery calcification and abnormal exercise test for coronary artery disease in asymptomatic men. *Circulation* 1980; 62:1196-203.

[38] Yeung AC, Barry J, Orav J et al. Effect of asymptomatic ischemia on long-term prognosis in chronic stable coronary disease. *Circulation* 1991; 83:1598-604.

[39] Fazzini PF, Prati PL, Rovelli F et al. Epidemiology of silent myocardial ischemia in asymptomatic middle-aged men (the ECIS Project). *Am J Cardiol* 1993; 72:1383-8.

[40] Froehicher VF, Thompson AJ, Longo MR Jr et al. Value of exercise testing for screening asymptomatic men for latent coronary artery disease. *Prog Cardiovasc Dis* 1976; 18:265-76.

[41] Thaulow E, Erikssen J, Sandik L et al. Initial clinical presentation of cardiac disease in asymptomatic men with silent myocardial ischemia and angiographically documented coronary artery disease: the Oslo ischemic study. *Am J Cardiol* 1993; 72:629-33.

[42] Langer A, Freeman MR, Josse RG, et al. Detection of silent myocardial ischemia in diabetes mellitus. *Am J Cardiol* 1991; 67:1073-8.

[43] Naka M, Hiramatsu K, Aizawa T et al. Silent myocardial ischemia in patients with non-insulin-dependent diabetes mellitus as judged by treadmill exercise testing and coronary angiography. *Am Heart J* 1992; 123:46-53.

[44] Multiple Risk Factor Intervention Trial Research Group. Exercise electrocardiogram and coronary heart disease mortality in the Multiple Risk Factor Intervention Trial. *Am J Cardiol* 1985; 55:16-24.

[45]   Dweck M, Campbell IW, Miller D et al. Clinical aspects of silent myocardial ischaemia: with particular reference to diabetes mellitus. *Vasc Health Risk Manag.* 2010; 6: 635–656.

[46]   Scognamiglio R, Negut C, Ramondo A et al. Detection of coronary artery disease in asymptomatic patients with Type 2 diabetes mellitus. *J Am Coll Cardiol* 2006; 47:65.

[47]   Zellweger MJ, Hachamovitch R, Kang X et al. Prognostic relevance of symptoms versus objective evidence of coronary artery disease in diabetic patients. *Eur Heart J* 2004; 25:543-50.

[48]   Rajagopalan N, Miller TD, Hodge DO et al. Identifying high-risk asymptomatic diabetic patients who are candidates for screening stress single photon emission computed tomography imaging. *J Am Coll Cardiol* 2005; 45:43-9.

[49]   Belch JJF, Topol EJ, Agnelli G et al. Critical issues in peripheral arterial disease detection and management: a call to action. *Arch Intern Med* 2003; 163:884-92.

[50]   Hertzer NR , Beven EG , Young JR et al. Coronary artery disease in peripheral vascular patients: A classification of 1000 coronary angiograms and results of surgical management. *Ann Surg* 1984; 199:223-33.

[51]   O'Sullivan JJ, Conroy RM, MacDonald K et al. Silent ischemia in diabetic men with autonomic neuropathy. *Br Heart J* 1991;66:313-5.

[52]   Niakan E, Harati Y, Rolak LA et al. Silent myocardial infarction and diabetic cardiovascular autonomic neuropathy. *Arch Intern Med* 1986; 146:2229-30.

[53]   Ma RC , So WY, Yang X et al. Erectile dysfunction predicts coronary heart disease in type 2 diabetics. *J Am Coll Cardiol* 2008; 51:2045-50.

[54]   Gazzaruso C, Giordanetti S, De Amici E et al. Relationship between erectile dysfunction and silent myocardial ischemia in apparently uncomplicated type 2 diabetic patients. *Circulation* 2004; 110:22-6.

[55]   Kannel WB, Feinleib M. Natural history of angina pectoris in the Framingham study. Prognosis and survival. *Am J Cardiol* 1972; 29:154–163.

[56]   Reunanen A, Suhonen O, Aromaa A, Knekt P, Pyorala K. Incidence of different manifestations of coronary heart disease in middle-aged Finnish men and women. *Acta Med Scand* 1985; 218:19–26.

[57]   Lerner DJ, Kannel WB. Patterns of coronary heart disease morbidity and mortality in the sexes: a 26-year follow-up of the Framingham population. *Am Heart J* 1986; 111:383–390.

[58]   Philpott S, Boynton PM, Feder G, Hemingway H. Gender differences in descriptions of angina symptoms and health problems immediately prior to angiography: the ACRE study. Appropriateness of Coronary Revascularisation study. *Soc Sci Med* 2001;52:1565–1575.

[59]   Daly CA, Clemens F, Sendon JL, Tavazzi L, Boersma E, Danchin N, Delahaye F, Gitt A, Julian D, Mulcahy D, Ruzyllo W, Thygesen K, Verheugt F, Fox KM; Euro Heart Survey Investigators. Gender differences in the management and clinical outcome of stable angina. *Circulation* 2006; 113:467–469.

[60] Kurita A, Takase B, Uehata A, Maruyama T, Nishioka T, Sugahara H et al. Painless myocardial ischemia in elderly patients compared with middle-aged patients and its relation to treadmill testing and coronary hemodynamic. *Clin Cardiol* 1991; 14:886–890.

[61] Vasilomanolakis EC. Geriatric cardiology: when exercise stress testing is justified. *Geriatrics* 1985; 40:47–50–53–4, 57.

[62] Noto TJ Jr, Johnson LW, Krone R, Weaver WF, Clark DA, Kramer JR Jr et al. Cardiac catheterization 1990: a report of the Registry of the Society for Cardiac Angiography and Interventions (SCAandI). *Catheter Cardiovasc Diagn* 1991; 24:75–83.

[63] Mehran R, Aymong ED, Nikolsky E, Lasic Z, Iakovou I, Fahy M et al. A simple risk score for prediction of contrast-induced nephropathy after percutaneous coronary intervention: development and initial validation. *J Am Coll Cardiol* 2004; 44:1393–1399.

In: Current Issues in the Management of Stable Ischemic Heart … ISBN: 978-1-62417-203-8
Editor: Mukesh Singh © 2013 Nova Science Publishers, Inc.

Chapter III

Use of Stress Testing Prior to PCI in Stable Coronary Artery Disease

Rahul Mehrotra, Mansi Kaushik and Ravi R. Kasliwal[*]
Medanta- The Medicity, Gurgaon, India

Abstract

Chronic stable angina is one of the myriad clinical syndromes associated with atherosclerotic CAD. Effective and timely intervention for chronic angina relies on early and systematic evaluation of the patients presenting with or suspected of having chronic angina. Stress tests play a crucial role in the patients of chronic angina for diagnosis, risk stratification and guiding the treatment plan. A clear understanding of the various stress tests available, their efficacy and utility is thus essential for all cardiologists managing such patients. We discuss here the role of stress testing in the patients of chronic angina going for percutaneous coronary intervention.

Conflict of interest: None

Introduction

The burden of coronary artery disease (CAD) has assumed vast proportions globally. In-spite of the enormous progress made in the development of new diagnostic methods and effective treatment approaches, CAD and its sequelae remain one of the biggest killers of the modern times. Previously believed to affect only the underdeveloped countries, the scenario has changed widely and the epidemic is now raging across the developing countries as well. The increased CAD burden is largely a result of high prevalence of underlying risk factors

[*] Address for correspondence: Ravi R Kasliwal, MBBS, MD, DM (Cardiology). Chairman, Clinical and Preventive Cardiology, # 9, 3rd Floor, Medanta- The Medicity,Sector 38, Gurgaon, Haryana- 122001, India. Ph: +91-124-4141414; Fax: +91-124-4834111; Email: rrkasliwal@hotmail.com.

like metabolic syndrome, obesity, diabetes and dyslipidemia due to unhealthy diet and sedentary, stressful lifestyle.

The scourge of CAD has to be tackled by primordial, primary and secondary prevention approaches. Efforts are on for increasing awareness at the population level, enacting laws to curb the use of saturated fats and by promoting healthy lifestyle in general, by the governments and policymakers. Similarly strides have been made in understanding the pathophysiology of CAD, developing new drugs and effective Percutaneous and surgical techniques for treatment of coronary artery disease and its attendant complications.

Chronic stable angina is one of the myriad clinical syndromes associated with atherosclerotic CAD. Effective and timely intervention for chronic angina relies on early and systematic evaluation of the patients presenting with or suspected of having chronic angina. Stress tests play a crucial role in the patients of chronic angina for diagnosis, risk stratification and guiding the treatment plan. A clear understanding of the various stress tests available, their efficacy and utility is thus essential for all cardiologists managing such patients. We discuss here the role of stress testing in the patients of chronic angina going for percutaneous coronary intervention.

Pathophysiology of Chronic Stable Angina

Anginal pain is caused by hypoxia of the myocardial tissue, which most commonly is due to a shortage of blood flow to the myocardium in comparison to its requirements (myocardial ischemia) [1]. Myocardial ischemia is thus the result of myocardial blood supply-demand mismatch. While myocardial oxygen supply depends on coronary blood flow, arterial oxygen saturation and myocardial oxygen extraction, myocardial oxygen demand is determined by heart rate, contractility and myocardial stress (Figure 1). Since myocardium already has very high oxygen extraction at rest (>75%), it is usually the limitation in flow which is the cause of ischemia in times of increased demand. Atheromatous plaque in the epicardial coronary arteries drastically alters luminal cross-sectional area, increases arteriolar tone and is thus, the most common cause of stable angina seen in clinical practice.

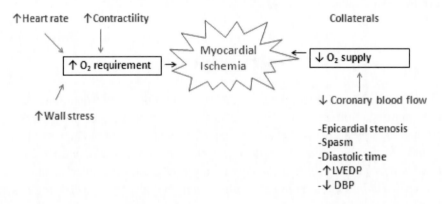

Figure 1. Pathophysiology of myocardial ischemia.

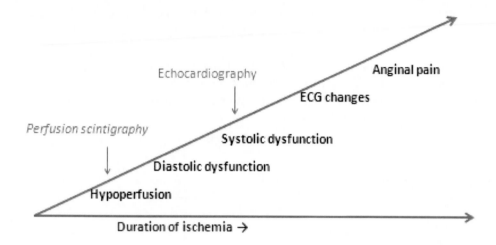

Figure 2. The cascade of events that occur following myocardial ischemia and the imaging modality used to detect them.

Table 1. Pretest probability of CAD by Age, Gender and Symptoms

Age (Yr)	Gender	Typical/Definite Angina Pectoris	Atypical/Probable Angina Pectoris	Non anginal Chest Pain	Asymptomatic
30-39	Men	Intermediate	Intermediate	Low	Very low
	Women	Intermediate	Very low	Very low	Very low
40-49	Men	High	Intermediate	Intermediate	Low
	Women	Intermediate	Low	Very low	Very low
50-59	Men	High	Intermediate	Intermediate	Low
	Women	Intermediate	Intermediate	Low	Very low
60-69	Men	High	Intermediate	Intermediate	Low
	Women	High	Intermediate	Intermediate	Low

(High, > 90%; intermediate, 10-90%; low, <10%; and very low < 5%).

Once Myocardial ischemia occurs, it induces sympathetic activation which through a variety of mechanisms like increased coronary vasoconstriction and oxygen consumption, further worsens ischemia and a series of events is initiated referred to as the "*ischemic cascade*" (Figure 2). Ischemic cascade is characterized by events like metabolic abnormalities due to tissue hypoxia, perfusion mismatch, diastolic dysfunction, systolic dysfunction electrocardiographic changes and finally, anginal pain [2, 3].

It is thus easy to understand that in patients with stable CAD, asymptomatic myocardial ischemia appears much before symptomatic ischemia [4]. This is also useful in understanding the sensitivity of various tests for detecting myocardial ischemia (see table 2). It is also useful to know that repetitive episodes of ischemia can lead to reversible myocardial contractile dysfunction called *stunning*. Similarly, recurrent myocardial ischemia and stunning for a longer period of time can lead to yet another form of reversible myocardial dysfunction known as *hibernation. Ischemic preconditioning,* which results in response to brief episodes of ischemia [5], is an endogenous adaptation for protection against myocardial ischemia.

Table 2. Sensitivity and specificity of different stress tests for detecting underlying coronary artery disease. These are approximate values since the results depend on the studies included and the patient groups studied

Diagnostic test	Sensitivity	specificity
Exercise electrocardiography	68%	77%
Exercise Echocardiography	85%	81%
Dobutamine Stress Echocardiography	81%	79%
Exercise SPECT	88%	72%
Pharmacological SPECT	90%	82%
CMR-Dobutamine stress	94%	90%

Coronary Artery Disease and Chronic Angina

As already discussed, the most common pathological substrate for stable CAD is atheromatous narrowing of coronary arteries. The normal vascular bed has the ability to increase blood flow up to 5-6 times in response to exercise by reduction in vascular resistance. This ability to reduce coronary vascular resistance and increase blood flow is impaired in a patient with atherosclerotic plaque in the epicardial vessels. With $\leq 40\%$ luminal obstruction, coronary flow in response to exercise is usually maintained. However, when luminal diameter reduction approaches 50%, coronary blood flow becomes inadequate to meet increased metabolic demand during exercise. With severe degrees of obstruction, coronary vascular resistance rises exponentially (almost three times between obstruction of 80% and 90%) [6]. Other factors which play a role in determination of ischemic threshold are - degree of development of collateral circulation, coronary vascular tone, transmural distribution of myocardial perfusion from sub endocardium to sub epicardium and platelet aggregation.

Although it is labeled as "stable", it is useful to remember that the threshold for angina may vary from time to time owing to several factors [7] and that the patients are always at risk of developing acute coronary syndrome (ACS). Data from Framingham heart study had shown that in the population with initial presentation of stable angina, 2 year incidence of non-fatal MI was 14.3% and 6.2%, whereas incidence of coronary heart disease (CHD) deaths was 5.5% and 3.8% in men and women respectively [8].

Diagnosis and Assessment of Chronic Angina

Within a population with chronic stable angina, the overall prognosis is quite variable from patient to patient and is dependent upon several factors related to baseline clinical condition, functional capacity and coronary anatomy. Therefore prognostic assessment becomes the integral part of management of patient with stable CAD. It is important to segregate patients with more severe forms of CAD who are potential candidates for revascularization (PCI or CABG) from those with less severe form of disease, who can do well on medical therapy alone, thereby avoiding unnecessary interventions in the latter group [9]. Therefore, stratification of patients into low, intermediate and high risk categories is a fundamental part of evaluation of patients of chronic stable angina.

The overall diagnostic assessment of a patient of stable angina is thus aimed at confirmation of diagnosis, risk stratification and evaluation of the efficacy of ongoing treatment. It involves clinical examination, laboratory tests and noninvasive / invasive cardiac investigations. However, even before selecting a patient for investigations, it is possible to triage the patients into different risk categories based on age, gender and the symptoms [10] (see table 1).

The patients with intermediate probability should proceed further to non-invasive stress testing while the patients with high probability of underlying CAD benefit most by going in for invasive testing followed by revascularization. The patients with very low or low probability need not undergo further evaluation and can safely be managed by medical therapy, including antidepressants. All the patients should also undergo laboratory tests aimed at identifying associated risk factors and co-morbid conditions like diabetes mellitus, dyslipidemia, renal disease etc.

Stress Testing in Chronic Stable Angina

The basic principle of stress testing is to induce myocardial ischemia by increasing cardiac work. The stressing modality can be either exercise, the most physiological mode, of pharmacological, with the use of drugs like dobutamine. Myocardial ischemia can be picked up by either electrocardiogram (ECG) or one of the imaging modalities {echocardiography, nuclear perfusion scintigraphy using single photon emission computed tomography (SPECT) or MRI}.

For the patients of chronic angina and intermediate pretest probability of CAD, who can exercise and have an interpretable resting ECG [2], Exercise stress testing is performed, while pharmacological stress testing is chosen for those who are unable to exercise due to any reason or have an ECG which is likely to interfere with the interpretation of ST-T changes. These are the patients with pre-excitation syndrome, those who are being paced, in presence of complete left bundle branch block (LBBB), ST segment depression of over 1mm, myocardial infarction within last two days, unstable angina, pericarditis, heart failure, severe aortic stenosis, severe uncontrolled lung disease, uncontrolled arrhythmia, uncontrolled hypertension, active cerebral ischemia or embolic phenomena, aortic dissection, myocarditis, endocarditis or any other unresolved acute medical condition.

Various stress tests have been in use and are described according to the methods used to induce and detect ischemia. The sensitivity of the various stress tests is however, different and is explained by the series of events in the ischemic cascade (see figure 2 and table 2). Stress tests not only detect ischemia but also can assess its extent and severity. Other information that can be obtained includes- functional capacity of the patient (exercise stress tests) and viability assessment (nuclear perfusion scintigraphy and dobutamine stress echo-cardiography).

Stress Testing and Percutaneous Coronary interventions (PCI)

Most patients of CAD and stable angina, who have suitable lesions and vessel anatomy amenable to PCI benefit greatly from the procedure. The aims of intervention are to allow relief from angina, improve functional capacity and prevent repeat intervention. The patients undergo the procedure through percutaneous approach, under local anesthesia and thus can safely be discharged after one or two days. However, not all patients of chronic angina should be subjected to invasive coronary angiography and not all candidates are suitable for the interventional procedure. Besides, there are risks involved due to its invasive nature. Careful selection of the patients for PCI is thus paramount for optimum benefit and minimizing risk. Non-invasive stress testing plays a pivotal role in this scenario and is widely recommended for this purpose.

According to the guidelines for PCI by American college of cardiology/American Heart Association and the society of cardio vascular angiography and intervention for patients with stable CAD, moderate to severe ischemia should be documented by non-invasive methods prior to coronary intervention. The most common method of documenting ischemia is by non-invasive stress testing. The patients who undergo stress testing prior to angioplasty have been shown to have lower in-hospital stay and a lower rate of future interventions [22]. Apart from confirming the diagnosis of CAD in a patient with stable angina, stress testing is also useful to assess the following parameters-(1) Documentation of extent and severity of ischemia; (2) Prognostication of patient with stable CAD; and (3) Assessment of myocardial viability.

Stress tests with imaging are superior to exercise electrocardiography in terms of their sensitivity of detection of obstructive coronary artery disease, ability to quantify the extent and severity of ischemia and also for localization of areas of ischemia. The patients who undergo stress testing can further be classified according to the result and not all candidates with a positive stress test are suitable for coronary angiography and intervention (table 3). The patients who have a low-risk stress test should be kept on optimal medical therapy whereas for patients who have intermediate or high risk stress test, an invasive strategy is advocated. However, in those candidates who have had coronary angiography done beforehand, but have intermediate severity lesions (50-70% stenosis), stress testing is useful in demonstrating the presence and severity of ischemia [11]. Therefore performing a stress test for selecting suitable candidates for PCI is of paramount value in managing patients of chronic angina. Several studies have demonstrated that for patients with stable CAD who underwent PCI with optimal therapy, outcome in terms of death and risk of future myocardial infarction did not differ from patients treated with optimal medical therapy alone [12-20].

Assessment of Prognosis

In addition to aiding in the diagnosis, stress testing also provides useful data for prognostication of patient with stable CAD. It has been shown that functional capacity as determined by exercise testing is one of the most important predictor of outcome regardless of the cause of termination of the exercise test (angina equivalent symptoms or fatigue). Each metabolic equivalent (MET) achieved in functional capacity is associated with a 12% increase in survival. Patients who achieve < 5 METs are at more than four fold higher risk of death compared to individuals who achieve > 10.7 METs [21].

Table 3. Approach to risk stratification after non-invasive stress testing

- Low-risk stress test (less than 1% annual cardiac mortality risk)
  - Treadmill score ≥ 5
  - Normal / small perfusion defect at rest or stress
  - Normal stress echo/ no change of limited resting wall motion during stress
- Intermediate-risk stress test (1-3% annual cardiac mortality risk)
  - Treadmill score -11 to less than 5
  - Resting LV dysfunction (LVEF 35-49%)
  - Limited ischemia on stress echocardiography, involving≤ 2 segments at high dose dobutamine
  - Moderate stress induced perfusion defect without LV cavity dilatation or lung uptake (of thallium-201)
- High-risk (>3% annual cardiac mortality risk)
  - Severe LV dysfunction at rest or post exercise (EF<35%)
  - Treadmill score ≤ -11
  - Echocardiographic wall motion abnormalities developing at low dose (up to 10mcg/kg/min) or at low heart rate(<120 beats/min), in >2 segments
  - Large, fixed perfusion defect with LV cavity dilatation or increased lung uptake (thallium 201)
  - Moderate stress induced perfusion defect with LV cavity dilatation or increased lung uptake (thallium 201)
  - Single large stress-induced perfusion defect or multiple perfusion defects of moderate size

Similarly, Duke treadmill score, that incorporates symptoms, ST-deviation and exercise capacity, indicates a 5 year morality rate of < 5% in patients with score >15 and 28% with a score of < -10 [22].

Additional prognostic data can be obtained by combing stress testing with myocardial imaging like nuclear perfusion or magnetic resonance imaging. On nuclear perfusion imaging, findings like single large stress induced perfusion defect or multiple moderate sized stress induced perfusion defects, large fixed defect with lung uptake of tracer or dilatation of ventricular cavity are indicative of increased annual mortality rate (table 3). Similarly, occurrence of ventricular systolic dysfunction during stress is one of the strongest makers of poor prognosis [10].

Assessment of Myocardial Viability

As is well known, prognosis in a patient with CAD largely depends on global left ventricular systolic function. Presence of an area of myocardial hibernation suggests that though diminished blood flow is enough to sustain viability, it is not adequate to maintain normal systolic function [23].

Observational studies have suggested that patients with substantial area of viable myocardium have better outcome in terms of regional and global myocardial function as well as long term survival compared to those with large areas of poor viability [24-25], if they undergo coronary intervention. Therefore assessment of myocardial viability is an essential prerequisite in patient with chronic CAD and LV dysfunction prior to coronary intervention.

Two non-invasive techniques detect different features of viable myocardium – perfusion imaging with Thallium–201 (SPECT) reflects cell membrane integrity while dobutamine echocardiography detects contractile reserve. A biphasic response with Dobutamine stress echocardiography is an indication of myocardial viability and a powerful predictor of functional recovery after PCI [26]. The number of viable segments is directly related to the long term favorable outcome in patients with CAD. Hence, non-invasive assessment of myocardial viability by stress test can be used to aid in the often difficult, decision making in patients with stable CAD and left ventricular dysfunction.

New imaging modalities like positron emission tomography (PET) and MRI have emerged in the last few years and have been combined with exercise and pharmacological stress to study the patients of coronary artery disease. Although the studies are few in number, there is evidence that these modalities have higher sensitivity and specificity for detecting CAD [28-30]. There is also emerging evidence of vasodilator stress myocardial perfusion imaging having prognostic value [31, 32].

Summary

Coronary artery disease and its sequel are one of the leading causes of morbidity and mortality worldwide. Chronic angina is one of the common syndromes of CAD arising due to myocardial ischemia. The diagnosis and management of chronic angina requires skillful understanding of the symptoms, their severity and systematic evaluation. Stress testing plays a crucial role in the triage of these patients and selecting the candidates suitable for coronary angiography and intervention. Stress testing also provides useful information like functional capacity and myocardial viability which not only has a bearing on long term prognosis, but also predicts recovery after revascularization. There is sufficient amount of outcome data available with the use of exercise ECG, exercise and pharmacological echocardiography and perfusion imaging using SPECT. The guidelines for management of patients with chronic angina and percutaneous coronary interventions also support the use of these stress tests in these patients. Technological advances in imaging coupled with emergence of new, more sensitive techniques of evaluation like stress MRI and PET scanning is making the field more accurate and exciting. Thus, physicians should be encouraged to properly utilize stress tests in patients of chronic angina before subjecting them to coronary interventions.

References

[1]   Frishman WH: Pharmacology of the Nitrates in angina pectoris. *Am J Cardiol 1985*; 56(17):81-131.

[2]   Messerli FH, Mancia G, Conti CR, Pepine CJ. Guidelines on the management of stable angina pectoris: executive summary: the task force on the management of stable angina pectoris of the European society of cardiology. *Eur Heart J.* 2006 Dec; 27(23):2902-3.

[3]   Conti CR, Bavry AA, Petersen JW. Silent Ischemia, clinical relevance. *J Am Coll Cardiol* 2012; 59:435-41.

[4]   Schang ST, Pepine CJ transient asymptomatic ST-segment depression during daily activity. *J Am Coll Cardiol* 1977; 39:396-402.

[5]   Tomai F, Crea F, chiariello L, Gioffre PA. Ischemic preconditioning in humans: models, mediators and clinical relevance. *Circulation* 1999; 100: 559-563.

[6]   Gould KL. Effect of coronary stenosis on coronary flow reserve and resistance. *J Am Coll Cardiol* 1974; 34:48-55.

[7]   Pupita G, Maseri A, Kaski JC, Galassi AR, Gavrielides S, Davies G et al. Myocardial ischemia caused by distal coronary artery contriction in stable angina pectori. N Engl J Med 1990; 323:314-520.

[8]   Kannel WB, Feinleib M. Natural history of angina pectoris in the Framingham study. Prognosis and survival. *Am J Cardiol* 1972; 29(2): 154-63.

[9]   Bassand J P, Hamn CW, Ardissino D, Boersma E, Budaj A, Fernandez-Aviles F, Fox KA, Hasdai D, Ohman EM, Wallentin L, Wijns W. Guidelines for the diagnosis and treatment of non- ST-segment elevation acute coronary syndromes. *Eur Heart J* 2007 Jul; 28(13):1598-600.

[10] Gibbons RJ, Balady GJ, Bricker JT Chaitman BR, Fletcher GF, Froelicher VF et al. ACC/AHA 2002 Guideline update for exercise testing: summary article. A report of the American college of Cardiology/American Heart Association task force on practice guidelines (committee to update the 1997 exercise testing guidelines). *J Am Coll Cardiol.* 2002; 40(8):1531-40.

[11] Ciaroni S, Bloch A, Hoffmann J L, Bettoni M, Fournet D. Prognostic value of dobutamine echocardiography in patients with intermediate coronary lesions at angiography. *Echocardiography* 2002; 19: 549-553.

[12] Boden WE, O' Rourke RA, Teo KK, et al. Optimal medical therapy with or without PCI for stable coronary disease. *N Engl J Med.* 2007; 356 (15): 1503-1516.

[13] Bucher HC, Hengstler P, Schindler C, Guyatt GH. Percutaneous transluminal coronary angioplasty versus medical treatment for non-acute coronary heart disease: a meta-analysis of randomised controlled trials. *BMJ.* 2000; 321 (7253): 73-77.

[14] Katritsis DG, Ioannidis JP. Percutaneous coronary intervention versus medical therapy in nonacute coronary artery disease. *Circulation.* 2005; 111 (22): 2906-2912.

[15] Folland ED, Hartigan PM, Parisi AF. Veterans Affairs ACME investigators. Percutaneous transluminal coronary angioplasty versus medical therapy for stable angina pectoris: outcomes for patients with double-vessel versus single-vessel coronary artery disease in a veterans affairs cooperative randomized trial. *J Am Coll Cardiol.* 1997, 29 (7): 1505-1511.

[16] Pitt B, Waters D, Brown WV, et al; Atorvastatin versus Revascularization Treatment Investigators. Aggressive lipid-lowering therapy compared with angioplasty in stable coronary artery disease. *N Engl J Med.* 1999; 341 (2): 70-76.

[17] Henderson RA, Pocock SJ, Clayton TC, et al, Seven year outcome in the RITA-2 trial: coronary angioplasty versus medical therapy. *J Am Coll Cardiol.* 2003; 42 (7): 1161-1170.

[18] Hueb W, Lopes NH, Gersh BJ, et al. Five-year follow-up of Medicine, Angioplasty, or Surgery Study (Mass II): a randomized controlled clinical trial of 3 therapeutic strategies for multivessel coronary artery disease. *Circulation.* 2007; 115 (9): 1082-1089.

[19] Hueb W, Soares PR, Gersh BJ, et al. The medicine, angioplasty, or surgery study (MASS-II): a randomized, controlled clinical trial of three therapeutic strategies for multivessel coronary artery disease: one year results. *J Am Coll Cardiol.* 2004; 43 (10): 1743-1751.

[20] Hueb W, Lopez BH, Gersh BJ, et al. Five-year follow up of Medicine, Angioplasty, or Surgery Study (MASS-II): a randomized controlled clinical trial of therapeutic strategies for multivessel coronary artery disease. *Circulation* 2007;115(9);1082-1089.

[21] Myers J, Prakash M, Froelicher V, Do D, Partington S, Atwood JE. Exercise Capacity and mortality among men referred for exercise testing. *N Eng J Med.* 2002; 346: 743-801.

[22] Show L J, Peterson E D, Show L K, Kesler K L, De Long E R, Harrell F E Jr Mahlbaier L H, Mark D M. Use of a prognostic treadmill score in identifying diagnostic coronary disease subgroup. *Circulation,* 1998; 98: 1622-1630.

[23] Grace AL; Dudley RA; Lucas FL; Malenka DJ; Hoff EV; Redburg RF; Frequency of stress testing to document ischemia prior to elective percutaneous coronary intervention JAMA. 2008; 300 (15): 1765-1773.

[24] Rahimtoola SH, The hibernating myocardium. *Am heart J* 1989; 117: 211-221.

[25] Box J J, Poldermans D, Elhendy A, et al. Improvement of left ventricular ejection fraction, heart failure symptoms and prognosis after revascularisation in patient with chronic coronary artery disease and viable myocardium detected by dobutamine stress echocardiography. *J Am Coll Cardiol.* 1999; 34: 163-169.

[26] Afridi I, Aroyburn PA, Panza JA, Oh JK, Zoghbi WA, Marwick TH. Myocardial viability during dobutamine echocardiography predicts survival in patients with coronary artery disease and severe left ventricular systolic function. *J Am Coll Cardiol* 1998; 32: 921-926.

[27] Afridi I, Kleiman NS, Raizner AE, Zoghibi WA, Dobutamine echocardiography in myocardial hibernation. Optimal dose and occuracy in predicting recovery of coronary angioplasty. *Circulation* 1995; 91: 663-70.

[28] Go RT, Marwick TH, MacIntyre WJ, et al. A prospective comparison of rubidium-82 PET and thallium-201 SPECT myocardial perfusion imaging utilizing a single dipyridamole stress in the diagnosis of coronary artery disease. *J Nucl Med* 1990; 31:1899-905.

[29] Tamaki N, Yonekura Y, Senda M et al. Value and limitation of stress thallium-201 single photon emission computed tomography: Comparison with N-13 ammonia positron tomography. *J Nucl Med* 1988; 29:1181-8.

[30] Pennell DJ. Cardiovascular Magnetic Resonance. *Circulation* 2010; 192:692-705.

[31] Yoshinaga K, Chow BJW, de Kemp RA, et al. what is the prognostic value with rubidium-82 perfusion positron emission tomography imaging? *J Am Coll Cardiol* 2006; 48:1029-39.

[32] Marwick TH, Shan K, Go RT, MacIntyre WJ, Lauer MS. Use of positron emission tomography for prediction of perioperative and late cardiac events before vascular surgery. *Am Heart J* 1995; 130:1196-202.

In: Current Issues in the Management of Stable Ischemic Heart … ISBN: 978-1-62417-203-8
Editor: Mukesh Singh © 2013 Nova Science Publishers, Inc.

Chapter IV

Medical Treatment Strategies for Stable Angina

Jawad M. Khan[*] and Lucy Duckworth

Department of Cardiology, City Hospital, Birmingham, UK

Abstract

This chapter focuses on the pharmacological management of stable angina. The different classes of drugs that provide prognostic benefit (anti-platelets, statins, angiotensin converting enzyme inhibitors and beta blockers) and symptomatic benefit (beta blockers, organic nitrates, calcium channel blockers and potassium channel openers) are discussed. Taking each class of drug in turn, we describe their mechanism of action, pharmacokinetics, clinical indications, evidence base and possible side effects. The newer agents, ivabradine (sinus node inhibitor) and ranolazine (late sodium current inhibitor), are discussed. Finally, we review specific aspects of the pharmacological management of angina in cardiac syndrome X and vasospastic angina in addition to diabetic, female and elderly patients.

Introduction

The treatment of stable angina aims to minimise or abolish symptoms and thus improve quality of life. It also aims to improve prognosis by preventing myocardial infarction and death. These aims can be achieved through a combination of patient education, risk factor modification, pharmacological therapy and the use of revascularisation in the form of percutaneous coronary intervention (PCI, angioplasty) or coronary artery bypass graft surgery (CABG).

[*] Address for correspondence: Dr Jawad M Khan, Consultant Interventional Cardiologist and Honorary Senior Clinical Lecturer, Department of Cardiology, City Hospital, Birmingham, UK.

The COURAGE trial [1] re-affirmed the effectiveness of optimal medical therapy (OMT) in improving symptoms and prognosis in patients with stable angina. When OMT was compared to OMT and PCI (with bare metal stents), the incidence of cardiac death and myocardial infarction (2.1% and 11.8% respectively) was similar in both groups [1]. However, symptom relief was greater in the OMT and PCI group [1]. The results indicated that all patients with stable angina should be treated initially with OMT reserving PCI for those who failed to achieve adequate symptom control. The additional benefit of coronary angiography is that it allows determination of disease severity that would benefit prognostically from coronary artery bypass surgery; even in asymptomatic patients. It is recognised that silent ischemia occurs in 0.4-1% of the general population but 10-20% of diabetics [2-5] and, hence, a symptom driven approach is less applicable especially in diabetics.

It is imperative to provide patients with good education with regards the nature of their condition and possible consequences of disease progression, providing motivation in order to modify risk factors and to be compliant with pharmacological therapy. Patients should be advised with regards to smoking cessation, adopting a healthy diet whilst taking regular exercise and optimising their weight.

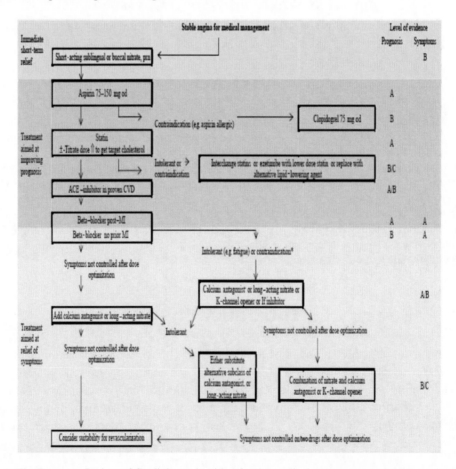

Figure 1. The European Society of Cardiology algorithm for the medical management of stable angina [6].

Co-existing conditions such as diabetes and hypertension should be optimised. Conditions that may be exacerbating symptoms, such as anaemia and hyperthyroidism, should be corrected.

Drugs that improve prognosis include anti platelet therapy, lipid lowering medication, angiotensin converting enzyme (ACE) inhibitors and beta blockers. Drugs that reduce the occurrence of angina with improved exercise tolerance include; beta blockers, organic nitrates, calcium channel blockers, and potassium channel openers such as nicorandil. Newer agents such as ivabradine and ranolazine have also been shown to be beneficial in providing symptom relief. As beta blockers improve prognosis and symptoms, they are first line therapy in patients with stable angina, with the aim being to optimise the dose as tolerated prior to adding additional agents for symptomatic relief (figure 1) [6].

Drugs with Prognostic Benefit

Drugs that improve prognosis include anti platelet therapy, lipid lowering medication, ACE inhibitors and beta blockers. They should be used in all patients with stable angina unless they are contraindicated or not tolerated.

Antiplatelet Therapy e.g. Aspirin, Clopidogrel, Dipyridamole, Prasugrel, Ticagrelor

Antiplatelet therapy has been shown to reduce the risk of coronary thrombosis in patients with stable coronary artery disease [7]. Aspirin remains the cornerstone of anti-platelet therapy in the context of stable angina. If aspirin is not tolerated, then clopidogrel is an effective alternative. Dipyridamole is not recommended in stable angina. Newer anti-platelet agents such as prasugrel (adenosine diphosphate receptor antagonist) and ticagrelor (platelet adenosine diphosphate P2Y12 receptor antagonist) are potent antiplatelet agents with rapid onset of action. However, at present they are not recommended for use in stable angina and their main indication is in ST elevation myocardial infarction (STEMI) where their rapid onset of action is beneficial. They can also be used following a stent thrombotic episode occurring whilst the patient is on clopidogrel (which suggests clopidogrel resistance).

Aspirin (Acetylsalicylic Acid)

Mechanism of Action
Aspirin irreversibly inhibits the enzyme cyclo-oxygenase type I (COX-1) which is involved in the conversion of arachidonic acid to thromboxane A2 (TXA2) which is a potent platelet aggregating agent. Hence, aspirin results in the inhibition of platelet aggregation. The inhibition of COX-1 by aspirin is irreversible and results in the reduced ability of platelets to aggregate throughout their lifespan. Aspirin also reduces expression of a cell surface receptor glycoprotein IIb/IIIa, and results in further inhibition of platelet aggregation (figure 2). Recovery from the anti-platelet effects of aspirin results from the production of new platelets

following cessation of aspirin therapy and, hence, recovery takes 7-10 days. The dose required to achieve platelet inhibition is much lower than that required for analgesia or the anti-inflammatory actions of aspirin [8].

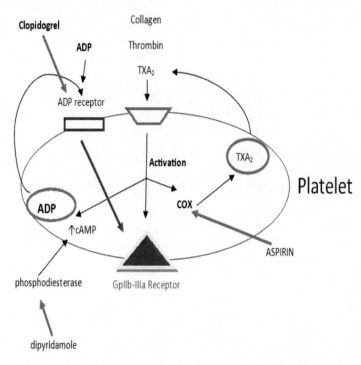

Figure 2. The mechanism of action of antiplatelet agents (ADP, adenosine diphosphate; TXA2, thromboxane A2; cAMP, cyclic adenosine monophosphate, COX, cyclo-oxygenase 1 enzyme; activate; , inhibit). The Glycoprotein IIb-IIIa receptor (GpIIb-IIIa receptor) is pivotal in platelet activation, aggregation (via fibrinogen) and adhesion to sub-endothelial proteins.

Pharmacokinetics

Aspirin is a weak organic acid and is well absorbed from the stomach and small intestine. It is metabolised in the tissues and blood to acetic acid and salicylate. The free salicylate and water soluble metabolites are excreted by the kidneys. The plasma half-life is between 2 and 19 hours after oral administration [8].

Clinical Indication and Evidence Base

The optimal dose of aspirin is 75 to 150 mg per day; above and below this dose the relative risk reduction afforded by aspirin reduces [9]. In the Swedish Angina Pectoris Aspirin Trial (SAPAT), there was a 34% reduction in myocardial infarction or cardiac death with an absolute risk reduction (ARR) of 1% per year when aspirin 75 mg once daily was compared to placebo in patients with stable angina [10]. Although the antiplatelet effects of aspirin do not increase with higher doses, the gastro-intestinal side effects do increase at higher doses [11]. Increasing the dose of aspirin from 75 to 160 mg once daily resulted in a 2 fold increase in peptic ulcer bleeding [12]. A further 2 fold increase was observed with increasing the dose to 325 mg per day [12]. The incidence of gastro-intestinal haemorrhage with aspirin at a dose less that 162.5 mg per day, was 2.3% versus 1.45% with placebo with a relative risk of 1.59 (95% confidence interval 1.4 to 1.81) [13].

Side Effects

Aspirin therapy can be associated with flushing, hypotension and tachycardia in addition to dizziness, tinnitus and headache. Gastrointestinal side effects such as nausea and dyspepsia can also occur. Compared to placebo, the increased risk of gastro-intestinal bleeding with low dose aspirin is less than 1% per year (2.3% versus 1.45% per year) [13]. A study by Chan et al in 2005 [14] showed the addition of esomeprazole (proton pump inhibitor) at 40mg per day to aspirin 80 mg once daily was better at preventing recurrent ulcer bleeding in patients with ulcers and vascular disease compared to switching to clopidogrel.

The risk of intracranial haemorrhage also increases with the use of aspirin [15], with an absolute risk of 1 per thousand patient years with aspirin more than 75 mg per day [16]. However, in patients with atherosclerotic vascular disease the reduction in ischaemic stroke offsets the increase risk of cerebral haemorrhage such that the net effect overall in terms of reducing stroke is beneficial [16]. Overall, the recommended dose of aspirin therapy is 75 mg once daily and at this dose it is an effective antiplatelet agent in addition to being well tolerated. Aspirin reduces the excretion of uric acid resulting in hyper-uricaemia and may contribute to the development of gout. A small proportion of individuals demonstrate salicylate intolerance developing an urticarial rash, swelling and headache. This is not a 'true allergy' but reflects an inability to metabolise even small amounts of aspirin.

Aspirin Resistance

The occurrence of cardiovascular events despite treatment with aspirin has led to interest in the resistance to the pharmacological effects of aspirin. However, there is no 'gold standard' method of assessing aspirin resistance and, therefore, identifying patients who may be aspirin resistant is difficult. The prevalence of resistance varies depending on the disease process and method of assessing platelet function [17]. In patients with previous stroke, aspirin resistance was associated with an 89% increase in recurrent cerebrovascular event rate over a two year period, compared to aspirin responders [17]. In the HOPE study [18], aspirin resistance was associated with a 3.5 fold increase in cardiovascular mortality and doubling of myocardial infarction. The cause of aspirin resistance is not known but is associated with intrinsic factors (variation in COX-1 structure preventing acetylation, thromboxane production by cells other than platelets, inducible COX-2 not inhibited by aspirin) and extrinsic factors (drug-drug interaction, tobacco smoking, inadequate dosing) [17].

Clopidogrel (ADP Receptor Antagonist)

Mechanism of Action

Clopidogrel inhibits platelet aggregation by binding irreversibly to the purinergic P2 receptor for adenosine diphosphate (ADP). This receptor is found on the surface of platelets and inhibition of this receptor results in reduced calcium mobilisation from intra-cellular stores within the platelet. In addition, the action of clopidogrel reduces the expression of the GP IIb/IIIa receptor on the surface of platelets (figure 2) [8].

Pharmacokinetics

Clopidogrel is well absorbed from the gastro-intestinal tract but is a pro drug and requires activation through liver metabolism to its active moiety. Due to the requirement for this metabolism, the onset of action of clopidogrel is slow and the maximum effect of clopidogrel occurs approximately 6 hours after a loading dose of 300 mg and approximately 2 hours after a 600 mg loading dose [19]. A higher loading dose has not been shown to be additionally beneficial [19]. Platelet inhibition is irreversible and recovery requires the formation of new platelets following cessation of clopidogrel therapy. Platelet function returns to normal 7 to 10 days after the last dose of clopidogrel. The half-life of the drug itself is approximately 7 hours [8].

Clinical Indication and Evidence Base

In the CAPRIE study [20], which assessed the benefit of clopidogrel versus aspirin (325 mg per day) in patients with previous myocardial infarction, previous stroke or peripheral vascular disease, clopidogrel was found to be more effective in preventing cardiovascular complications (absolute risk reduction of 0.51% per year; relative risk reduction of 8.7%, p value of 0.043). Clopidogrel had a slightly reduced occurrence of gastrointestinal haemorrhage compared to aspirin (1.99 versus 2.66%) [20]. In the CHARISMA trial [20], no added benefit in efficacy was seen by combining clopidogrel with aspirin compared to aspirin alone. The combination was associated with an increased risk of moderate and severe bleeding. Therefore, clopidogrel is recommended as an alternative to aspirin, if aspirin is not tolerated or contra-indicated, but combination therapy in stable angina is not recommended [21].

Side Effects

All antiplatelet agents carry the risk of bleeding although the risk associated with clopidogrel is low, conversely increased bruising is common. Gastrointestinal side effects can also occur such as dyspepsia, abdominal pain and diarrhoea. Additional side effects include headache, dizziness and paraesthesia. The combination of aspirin and clopidogrel is associated with 1% absolute increase in major, non-life threatening bleeding per year compared to aspirin alone [22]. It has also been associated with the occurrence of a widespread rash which can occur in up to 5.1% of individuals prompting discontinuation [22]. The rash resolves on cessation of clopidogrel but occasionally anti-histamines or steroids may be required until the rash resolves.

Clopidogrel Resistance

The increase in cardiovascular events despite clopidogrel therapy has prompted a search for clopidogrel resistance, however, there is no clear and accepted definition for clopidogrel resistance. Studies show a time and dose dependent response to clopidogrel therapy as assessed by ADP induced optical platelet aggregometry. [23-26]. In a study by Gurbel et al [23], 96 patients undergoing elective percutaneous coronary intervention (PCI or angioplasty) received clopidogrel 300mg loading followed by 75mg once daily. Clopidogrel resistance was defined as < 10% reduction in platelet aggregation in response to ADP compared to pretreatment levels. Clopidogrel resistance was seen in 63% of patients at 2 hours, 31% at 24 hours, 31% at 5 days and 15% at day 30 [23].

In a study by Matetzky et al [27], laboratory measures of clopidogrel resistance were correlated with clinical outcome, patients undergoing primary PCI for ST segment elevation myocardial infarction (STEMI) received 300mg loading dose followed by 75mg once daily for 3 months. Turbidometric analysis was undertaken following ADP and epinephrine stimulation to assess platelet function. Patients were divided in to four groups based on the degree of platelet inhibition caused by clopidogrel at day 6, compared to baseline platelet inhibition. At 6 months follow up, patients that exhibited clopidogrel resistance (i.e. the lowest quartile of platelet inhibition) experienced more cardiovascular events (stent thrombosis, myocardial infarction, recurrent ACS and peripheral arterial occlusion) [27].

The mechanisms responsible for clopidogrel resistance are multiple, including the reduced metabolism by Cytochrome P-450 P3A4 (resulting in variable conversion to the active metabolite), variable absorption of the pro-drug and increased excretion of the active metabolite [28]. P2Y12 receptor variability, increase in number of receptors, increased ADP release and up-regulation of additional pathways of platelet activation may also contribute.

Dipyridamole

Mechanism of Action

Dipyridamole inhibits the enzyme phosphodiesterase type V which is involved in the degradation of cyclic nucleotides. This results in an increase in intra-cellular concentrations of cyclic adenosine monophosphate (cAMP) within the platelets and reduces activation and expression of the glycoprotein IIb/IIIa receptor on the surface of platelets. This in turn results in inhibition of platelet aggregation (figure 2) [8].

Pharmacokinetics

Following the absorption from the gastro-intestinal tract dipyridamole is metabolised by the liver. It has a plasma half-life of approximately 12 hours [8].

Clinical Indication and Evidence Base

Dipyridamole is not recommended as an antiplatelet agent in the management of stable angina due to its weak antiplatelet effect. In addition, due to its vasodilating effect on the microvasculature it may worsen angina by resulting in redistribution of blood away from areas of the myocardium supplied by stenosed vessels (coronary steal phenomenon) [29].

Side Effects

Dipyridamole can cause dizziness and headaches in addition to flushing, hypotension and tachycardia. Gastro-intestinal side effects can also occur. Dipyridamole can also be associated with a hypersensitivity reaction manifesting as an urticarial rash, bronchospasm and angio-oedema [8].

Statin Therapy e.g. Atorvastatin, Simvastatin, Rosuvastatin, Pravastatin

Although there are a number of lipid lowering therapies available, the greatest evidence base exists for statin therapy, hence they are first line treatment.

Mechanism of Action

3-hydroxy-3-methylglutaryl coenzyme A (HMG-Co A) reductase inhibitors (statins) competitively inhibit the enzyme that catalyses the synthesis of cholesterol in the liver (figure 3). This is a rate limiting step and reduces hepatic cholesterol level. Increased clearance of circulating low density lipoprotein (LDL) cholesterol occurs due to up-regulation of hepatocyte surface LDL receptors resulting in a 25-50% reduction in LDL cholesterol. Hepatocyte very low density lipoprotein (VLDL) production is also reduced with consequent reduction in circulating triglycerides.

A small increase in high density lipoprotein (HDL) cholesterol is also observed. Rosuvastatin is the most potent of the statins, then atorvastatin, simvastatin and, lastly, pravastatin is least potent [8].

Pharmacokinetics

Statins are well absorbed from the gastro-intestinal tract. Atorvastatin has a very long half-life (32-36 hours) undergoing first pass liver metabolism in part to active derivatives. Simvastatin is a pro-drug with a half-life of 2 hours with poor bioavailability due to hepatic metabolism with only 5% of the active compound reaching the circulation [8]. Pravastatin has a half-life of 1-2 hours being eliminated by the kidneys [8]. Rosuvastatin has a long half-life of 20 hours but low oral bioavailability, being eliminated mainly in the bile [8]

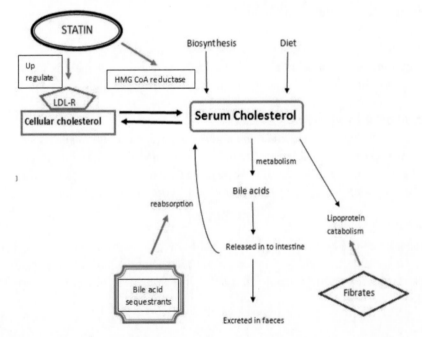

Figure 3. The mechanism of action of statins, bile acid sequestrants and fibrates (⟶, inhibition, up-regulate).

Clinical Indication and Evidence Base

Statin therapy has been shown to reduce the risk of cardiovascular complications in the context of primary and secondary prevention [30]. Statin therapy should be used in all patients with stable angina irrespective of their age and baseline cholesterol level. It has been shown to reduce cardiovascular events by approximately 30% with a reduction in mortality [31-33]. The Joint British Society (JBS-2) guidelines [34] recommend an optimal total serum cholesterol of less than 4 mmol/l (or 25% reduction from baseline, whichever is lower) with an LDL cholesterol of less than 2 mmol/l (or more than 30% reduction from baseline, whichever is lower). Statin therapy effectively lowers cholesterol [30] by inhibiting cholesterol synthesis, however, it has additional anti-inflammatory and anti-thrombotic effects [35, 36] which contribute to its reduction in cardiovascular events. Statins restore vascular endothelial function damaged by hypercholesterolaemia. They alter smooth muscle proliferation and migration, stabilising atherosclerotic plaques. Decreased plasma fibrinogen and increased fibrinolysis result in changes in haemostasis and inflammatory cell infiltration into atherosclerotic plaques is also reduced.

In patients with stable angina, pre-treatment prior to coronary angioplasty with 40 mg of Atorvastatin compared to placebo, reduced procedural myocardial injury (as assessed by biochemical markers) [37]. In patients who are intolerant to statin therapy then fibrates, nicotinic acid and ezetimibe may be used, although they are associated much less evidence of benefit [1, 38]. A meta-analysis undertaken in 2005 by Studer et al [39], showed no reduction in mortality with fibrates, resins or niacin. The latest evidence supports the use of simvastatin 40 mg once daily, pravastatin 40 mg once daily and atorvastatin 10 mg once daily [35, 36]. Increased dose of atorvastatin (80 mg once daily) has been shown to reduce the risk of cardiovascular events compared to atorvastatin 10 mg or simvastatin 24 mg in patients with stable angina [40, 41] but this was at the expense of a 6 fold increase in liver enzymes (0.2 to1.2%: p< 0.001) but no significant increase in myalgia [40].

Side Effects

Statin therapy is generally well tolerated but skeletal muscle side effects (myalgia, elevated creatine kinase and rarely rabdomyolisis) can occur. Baseline liver function tests ought to be measured and monitored after initiation of therapy. Although statin therapy, in addition to fibrates, can be used in patients with severe hyperlipidaemia, there is a significantly increased risk of associated myopathy and this combination ought to be used with caution. If combination therapy is required then fenofibrate appears to be the best tolerated [42]. Increasingly, statin therapy is used alongside ezetimibe which reduces cholesterol absorption (approximately 50%) and this combination is well tolerated [8]. Although this combination does provide significant reductions in cholesterol level the effects on morbidity and mortality have not yet been documented. In statin intolerant patients, ezetimibe can be given alone resulting in a 15% reduction in total cholesterol and 20% in LDL cholesterol [8]. When used in combination with low dose statins, the combination is as effective as three incremental doubling doses of statins [8].

Angiotensin Converting Enzyme (ACE) Inhibitors, e.g. Ramipril, Lisinopril, Perindopril, Enalapril and Captopril

Mechanism of Action

ACE inhibitors are competitive inhibitors of the plasma angiotensin converting enzyme (ACE) which reduces the level of circulating angiotensin II and the release of aldosterone. Angiotensin II is involved in the development of arterial remodelling and left ventricular hypertrophy in hypertension. Thus, ACE inhibitors result in arterial and venous dilatation and the reduction in aldosterone production also results in reduced salt and water retention by the kidneys. Both of the mechanisms result in reduction in blood pressure. ACE inhibitors arrest or reduce the processes that lead to atherosclerosis. Chronic overexpression of tissue angiotensin converting enzyme in coronary artery disease disrupts the angiotensin II/bradykinin balance resulting in endothelial dysfunction. ACE inhibitors reduce production of angiotensin II, which prevents vasoconstriction, reducing adhesion molecules and growth factors, decreasing oxidative stress and preventing apoptosis. A reduction in degradation of bradykinin raises levels of this kinin, leading to vasodilation and an anti-apoptotic action (figure 4) [8].

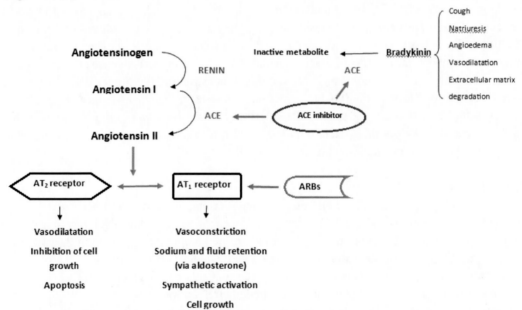

Figure 4. The mechanism of action of ACE inhibitors and angiotensin receptor blockers (ARBs) (inhibition; activation; ACE, angiotensin converting enzyme).

Pharmacokinetics

Active forms of ACE inhibitors are poorly absorbed from the gastrointestinal tract due to being polar and, therefore, many ACE inhibitors are given as pro drugs being converted in the liver to the active moiety e.g. ramipril is converted in the liver to ramiprilat (which is an active compound). ACE inhibitors, such as lisinopril and captopril, are well absorbed from the gastrointestinal tract as active molecules. Plasma half-life varies being approximately 2 hours for drugs such as captopril and ramiprilat, being 30 to 35 hours for the active metabolites of perindopril and enalapril [8].

Clinical Indication and Evidence Base

Although ACE inhibitors are used widely in the treatment of hypertension and heart failure, they have a beneficial effect in the context of stable coronary artery disease even in the absence of heart failure or hypertension. Ramipril and perindopril have been shown to reduce morbidity and mortality in moderate to high risk patients [43, 44]. In the HOPE study (Heart Outcomes Prevention Evaluation Study) [44], patients 55 years of age or older with previous cardiovascular event or at least one cardiovascular risk factor or diabetes, were randomised to ramipril versus placebo. Ramipril lowered the risk of combined primary outcome by 25%, with a reduction in myocardial infarction by 22%, stroke by 33% and cardiovascular death by 37% [44]. There was a total reduction in mortality of 24% with a 17% reduction in the need for revascularisation and a 24% reduction in the development of overt nephropathy [44]. These reductions were seen over a period of 4.5 years. Although there was a reduction in blood pressure with ramipril, after adjustment for this, there was still a reduction in primary outcome by 25% (p = 0.0004) [44].

In the EUROPA study [43], patients with stable coronary artery disease were randomised to perindopril versus placebo over a period of 4.2 years. Treatment with perindopril resulted in a 20% relative risk reduction in primary endpoints which was a composite of cardiovascular death, non-fatal myocardial infarction and cardiac arrest with successful resuscitation (p valve of 0.0003) [43]. There was also a 14% reduction in myocardial infarction, total mortality, unstable angina and cardiac arrest (p=0.0009) [43]. There was a 24% reduction in fatal and non-fatal myocardial infarction (p value less than 0.001) and a 39% reduction in hospital admission for heart failure (p=0.002) [43]. Studies have shown that higher the dose of ACE inhibitor, the greater the prognostic benefit and doses of 10 mg of ramipril and 8 mg of perindopril are recommended, if tolerated. If ACE inhibitors are not tolerated, then angiotensin receptor blockers can be used.

Side Effects

Accumulation of kinins in the lungs results in a persistent dry cough in 10 to 30% of individuals taking ACE inhibitors. The side effect may develop many months after commencing ACE inhibitor therapy and is more common in female patients [8].

ACE inhibition can result in reduced renal perfusion due to reduced angiotensin mediated arterial vasoconstriction of the efferent glomerular arterioles which maintains glomerular perfusion pressure. This can be especially severe in individuals who have bilateral renal artery stenosis and can result in rapid deterioration in renal function. Routine monitoring of renal function prior to and seven days after each incremental dose increase is recommended [8].

The vasodilating effects of ACE inhibitors can result in postural hypotension which can be a particular problem after first dose initiation.

ACE inhibitors can cause nausea, vomiting and dyspepsia in addition to a disturbance in taste and rash. Angioedema can also occur with the use of ACE inhibitors and this is more likely to occur in individuals of African or Afro Caribbean origin [8]. ACE inhibitors are teratogenic and should be avoided in female patients of childbearing age. If ACE inhibitors are not tolerated then angiotensin receptor blockers (ARBs) are a useful alternative [8].

Angiotensin Receptor Antagonists e.g. Losartan, Valsartan and Candesartan

Mechanism of Action

Angiotensin receptor antagonists or blockers (ARBs) work selectively on the angiotensin 1 receptor (AT1), which is found in the heart, lungs, kidneys, brain, adrenal cortex and blood vessels. Acting through the AT1 receptor, Angiotensin II results in vasoconstriction , aldosterone release (resulting in salt and water retention), sympathetic stimulation and cell growth and proliferation (figure 4). Kinin degradation is not affected by angiotensin receptor antagonists [8].

Pharmacokinetics

Losartan is well absorbed from the gastro-intestinal tract but undergoes extensive first pass metabolism. Losartan is a pro drug being metabolised in the liver to its active component with a half-life of between 9 and 12 hours [8]. It is eliminated by metabolism and renal excretion. Although losartan is a competitive antagonist at the AT1 receptor, its active metabolite is a non-competitive antagonist. Valsartan is not well absorbed from the gastro-intestinal tract. It has a half-life of between 5 to 7 hours and is metabolised by the liver [8].

Clinical Indication and Evidence Base

The effects of angiotensin receptor antagonist treatment, in the context of ischaemic heart disease, have been less well studied compared to ACE inhibitors. Valsartan was found to be as effective as captopril in post myocardial infarction patients with heart failure in the VALIANT study [45]. In the context of normal left ventricular systolic function, CHARM-Preserved study [46], candesartan was found to have no significant benefit compared to placebo. Thus, although ACE inhibitors are indicated in the management of patients with stable angina, angiotensin receptor blockers are only recommended in the context of stable angina with patients having concomitant heart failure, hypertension or diabetic renal dysfunction.

Side Effects

In comparison to ACE inhibitors, there is a low incidence of cough and, although angioedema can occur, this side effect is rare with angiotensin receptor antagonists. Additional side effects of ARBs include myalgia and arthralgia. Headache, dizziness and fatigue can also occur.

Beta Adrenoreceptor Antagonist (Beta Blockers) e.g. Atenolol, Metoprolol, Bisoprolol, Propanolol, Nebivolol, Carvedilol and Labetalol

As beta blockers provide both symptomatic and prognostic benefit, they are first line therapy in the management of stable angina.

Mechanism of Action

Beta blockers are competitive antagonists of catecholamines at beta adrenoreceptors. Reducing the generation of intra-cellular cyclic AMP through blocking cardiac Beta 1 adrenoreceptors results in the following [8]:

- A reduction in heart rate, particularly during exercise, achieved through inhibition of the If pacemaker current in the sino-atrial node (SAN). At any particular level of exertion, the corresponding heart rate is reduced.
- Reduced force of cardiac contraction.
- Reduction in blood pressure which is in part due to reduced renin release from the kidneys (renin leads to the synthesis of angiotensin II which is a potent vasoconstrictor).

The consequence of these changes is a reduced oxygen demand of the myocardium. As the myocardial perfusion is largely during diastole due to systolic compression of intra-myocardial vessels, the lengthening of diastole by the reduction in heart rate is additionally beneficial and results in improved myocardial blood flow.

Beta Adrenoreceptor Cardio-selectivity

Non selective beta blockers, such as propranolol, act equally on beta 1 and beta 2 adrenoreceptors. Cardioselective beta blockers (e.g. atenolol, metoprolol and bisoprolol) act selectively on beta 1 adrenoreceptors in the heart. However, this selectivity is reduced at higher doses producing greater beta 2 adrenoreceptor blockade [8].

Intrinsic Sympathomimetic Activity

Some beta blockers (e.g. pindolol) act as non-selective beta blockers but are also able to act as a partial agonist; resulting in a lower reduction in heart rate associated with their use. Therefore, they are less likely to result in beta blocker induced bradycardia [8].

Vasodilating Beta Blockers

Pure adrenoreceptor blockers do not result in vasodilatation and, in fact, reflex vasoconstriction can occur mediated by a fall in cardiac output stimulating alpha 1 adrenoreceptors. Combined alpha 1 adrenoreceptor and beta blockers (e.g. carvedilol and labetalol) or beta blockers that increase endothelial nitric oxide production (e.g. nebivolol) do result in vasodilatation [8].

Pharmacokinetics

Soluble (hydrophilic) beta blockers (e.g. pindolol and celiprolol) are incompletely absorbed from the gastro-intestinal tract and undergo limited first passed metabolism. They are subsequently eliminated through renal excretion. The half-life of hydrophilic beta blockers is longer than lipophilic beta blockers. Lipophilic beta blockers (e.g. propanolol and metoprolol) are well absorbed from the gastro-intestinal tract but undergo extensive first passed metabolism with limited bioavailability (10-30%) [8]. Consequently, plasma levels are variable and dose titration is required to achieve optimal clinical effect. Most lipophilic beta blockers have short half-lives (e.g. propanolol half live of 4 hours, metoprolol 3-10 hours) but modified release formulations are available which prolong their duration of action [8].

Clinical Indication and Evidence Base

In addition to improving symptoms, beta blockers also have prognostic benefit. They have been shown to improve prognosis in patients with heart failure [47] and in patients with previous myocardial infarction [48]. In the MERIT-HF study [47], patients with heart failure (New York Heart Association class II to IV) with a left ventricular ejection fraction of less than 44% on optimal medical therapy were randomised to metoprolol versus placebo. There was a 34% reduction in mortality, 41% reduction in sudden death and a 49% reduction in mortality due to progressive heart failure in the group treated with metoprolol [49]. In the CIBIS-II trial [50], patients with impaired left ventricular systolic function of 35% or less in class III or IV heart failure, were randomised to bisoprolol versus placebo in addition to optimal medical therapy. Bisoprolol treatment was associated with a significant reduction in all-cause mortality (11.8% with bisoprolol versus 17.3% with placebo) [50]. Similar beneficial effects were seen with carvedilol [51].

The APSIS [52] and TIBET [53] studies compared metoprolol with verapamil, and atenolol with nifedipine, respectively. Although there was no significant difference in outcomes between these study groups, the overall results showed excellent prognosis in the context of stable angina. The ASIST trial compared atenolol with placebo and showed a reduction in endpoints with the use of atenolol [51].

Side Effects

Beta 1 Adrenoreceptor Blockade

In the context of pre-existing severely impaired left ventricular systolic function, high sympathetic nervous activity is required to maintain cardiac output. High doses of beta blockers can, therefore, precipitate acute decompensation resulting in pulmonary oedema. Paradoxically, the use of low doses with gradual up-titration, in the context of compensated severely impaired left ventricular systolic function, is beneficial. The reduction in cardiac output caused by beta blockers can also exacerbate peripheral vascular disease or worsen Raynaud's phenomenon. The reduction in heart rate may be excessive, resulting in symptomatic bradycardia, fatigue and lethargy.

Beta 2 Adrenoreceptor Blockade

Blockade of beta 2 adrenoreceptors can result in bronchospasm in patients with asthma and chronic obstructive pulmonary disease (COPD) with reversibility.

If no significant reversibility is present with COPD then beta blockers are usually well tolerated. Cardio-selective beta blockers are preferred in patient with COPD without reversibility and, whether cardio-selective or not, beta blockers are contra-indicated in asthmatics [8].

Non selective beta adrenoreceptor blockers may prolong hypoglycaemia in diabetics treated with oral hypoglycaemic agents or insulin through inhibiting gluconeogenesis. Gluconeogenesis in the liver is dependent on beta 2 adrenoreceptors. The autonomic response that alerts diabetic individuals to the onset of hypoglycaemia can also be blunted by beta blockers and, therefore, they should be used in caution in patients who are prone to hypoglycaemia [8].

Central Nervous System Effects

Central nervous system effects are more common with lipophilic beta blockers (metoprolol, propranolol) which readily cross the blood brain barrier and can result in sleep disturbance, vivid dreams and hallucinations [8]. Lack of concentration through fatigue may also occur [8].

Effects of Lipid Profile

Most beta blockers result in elevation of triglyceride levels and reduction in high density lipoprotein cholesterol.

These changes can result in accelerated atherosclerosis.

Sudden Withdrawal Syndrome

Long term treatment with beta blockers results in up regulation of beta adrenoreceptors making the heart more sensitive to the effect of circulatory catecholamines. Sudden cessation of beta blockade results in reflex tachycardia which can precipitate symptoms of ischaemic heart disease resulting in the development of unstable angina or even myocardial infarction [8].

Drugs Used for Symptomatic Relief of Stable Angina

Drugs that reduce the occurrence of angina with improved effort tolerance include beta blockers, nitrates, calcium channel blockers, and potassium channel openers such as nicorandil.

New agents such as ivabradine (sinus node inhibitor) and ranolazine (late sodium current inhibitor) have also been shown to be beneficial. Beta blockers are first line therapy with optimisation of the dose prior to the addition of other anti-anginal therapy (figure 5).

Organic Nitrates e.g. Glyceryl Trinitrate, Isosorbide Dinitrate, Isosorbide Mononitrate

Mechanism of Action

Organic nitrates mimic the effects of endogenous nitric oxide resulting in vascular smooth muscle relaxation and vasodilatation. Enzyme degradation of nitrates results in nitric oxide which is converted in the vascular endothelium to nitrosothiols. Nitrosothiols result in the production of cyclic guanosine monophosphate (cGMP), through activating guanylyl cyclase (figure 6).

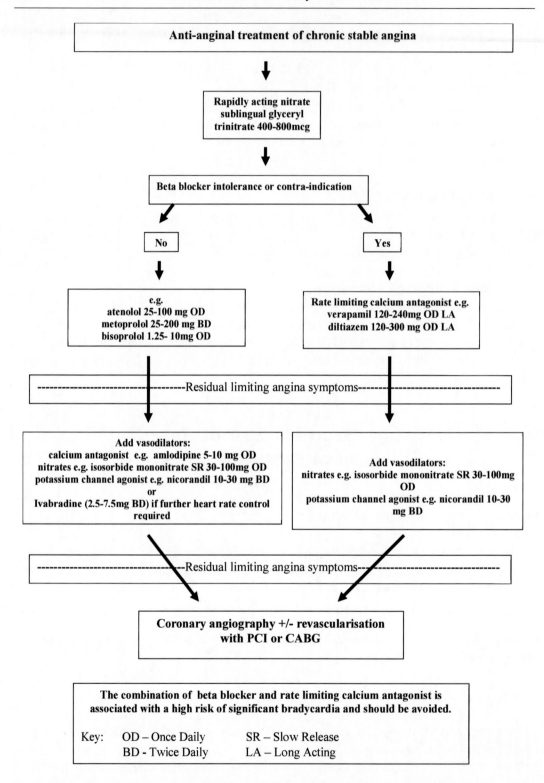

Figure 5. The stepwise increase in anti-anginal therapy to achieve symptomatic relief of angina.

This results in reduced availability of intra-cellular calcium and consequent smooth muscle relaxation and vasodilatation. This vasodilatation occurs in the coronary arteries resulting in increased blood flow through collateral vessels and the relief of coronary artery vasospasm. Vasodilatation also occurs in venous capacitance vessels. Reduced venous return to the heart results in reduced left ventricular filling pressure, reduced ventricular wall tension and hence, myocardial oxygen demand is reduced. Arterial vasodilation also reduces afterload reducing resistance to left ventricular emptying. The reduced cardiac work results in a reduction in myocardial oxygen demand [8].

Pharmacokinetics

Although glyceryl trinitrate (GTN) is well absorbed from the gastro-intestinal tract, it is a largely inactivated by first past metabolism. Hence glyceryl trinitrate is either given intravenously, trans-dermally, trans-buccal or sublingually.

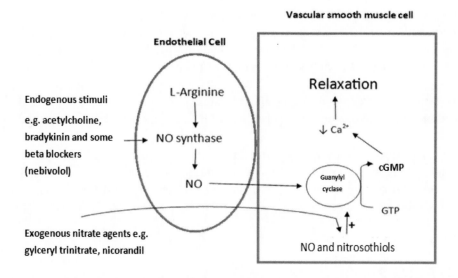

Figure 6. The mechanism of action of organic nitrates, nicorandil and nebivolol (Ca2+, calcium ion; cGMP, cyclic guanosine monophosphate; GTP, guanosine triphosphate; NO, nitric oxide).

Isosorbide dinitrate (ISDN) also undergoes extensive first passed metabolism with a short duration of action (0.5 to 2 hours). Isosorbide mononitrate (ISMN) has a longer plasma half-life (3 to 7 hours) and does not undergo first pass metabolism. Modified release preparations of isosorbide dinitrate results in a more prolonged duration of action with a longer half-life [8].

Clinical Indication and Evidence Base

Sublingual glyceryl trinitrate provides rapid symptom relief during attacks of exertion related angina and can, when used prophylactically, improve effort tolerance. Although they have rapid onset of action their effects are short lived (typically 20 minutes). Long acting nitrates such as isosorbide mononitrate or GTN patches reduce the frequency and severity of angina episodes. However, continued uninterrupted use of nitrates results in tolerance and, therefore, a nitrate free interval each day is advised to preserve the therapeutic effect of nitrates. Patients who use GTN patches should remove their patches at night time, however, rebound angina or reduced angina threshold may occur.

Long acting nitrates reduce the frequency and severity of angina attacks with an increase in exercise tolerance [55]. However, studies following myocardial infarction have failed to show a prognostic benefit [56].

Side Effects

Postural hypotension and dizziness can result from the vasodilatation. In some instances, this can result in reflex tachycardia and syncope. Arterial vasodilatation can result in flushing and headache. Sustained high plasma levels of nitrates can result in the development of tolerance.

The cause of tolerance is not well understood and may be related to the production of oxygen free radicals which result in nitric oxide breakdown. Activation of the renin angiotensin aldosterone system (RAAS) and synthetic nervous system (SNS), in response to hypotension, may also counteract the vasodilating actions of organic nitrates [8]. Conversely, co-administration of ACE inhibitors , angiotensin receptor blockers or hydralazine may reduce the occurrence of nitrate tolerance by impairing the formation of super oxides [8]. Tolerance can be avoided by introducing a nitrate free period for several hours during each day.

This can be achieved by removing nitrate patches at night time or by giving doses of isosorbide mono or dinitrate during the daytime with no dosage towards the evening or night time.

Long acting preparations given first thing in the morning will allow plasma nitrate concentrations to reduce overnight and this also reduces the occurrence of tolerance [8]. It is important to advise patients that GTN tablets decay when exposed to air and opened containers should be discarded within 3 months. The spray formulations of GTN are stable [8].

Calcium Channel Blockers e.g. Diltiazem, Verapamil, Amlodipine and Nifedipine

Mechanism of Action

Calcium channel blockers act by reducing calcium influx through voltage operated L-type calcium channels (figure 7). This results in the following action [8]:

1   Coronary dilatation. This is particularly useful in patients who have coronary vasospasm.
2   Arteriolar dilatation. Dihydropyridine calcium channel blockers (e.g. nifedipine and amlodipine) are potent vasodilators reducing peripheral resistance and reducing blood pressure. This reduces left ventricular work and consequently myocardial oxygen demand. Short acting dihydropyridines (e.g. nifedipine) result in reflex sympathetic nervous system activation leading to tachycardia in response to the reduction in blood pressure and are not recommended in the treatment of ischaemic heart disease. Modified release preparations of short acting dihydropyridines

(nifedipine retard or mr) result in a more gradual reduction in blood pressure with little reflex tachycardia. Similarly, longer acting agents (amlodipine) cause little tachycardia.

3   Negative chronotropic (heart rate) effect. Non dihydropyridine calcium channel blockers, such as verapamil and diltiazem, result in slowing of the heart rate due to their effects on the sino-atrial node but also on the atrio- ventricular node. They also blunt the rise in heart rate related to exercise. Therefore, although verapamil and diltiazem also result in vasodilatation, there is no reflex tachycardia.

4.   Negative inotropic effect. Most calcium channel blockers are negatively inotropic (reduce the strength of cardiac contraction) and this is a particular problem with verapamil. Amlodipine has no significant negative inotropic effects.

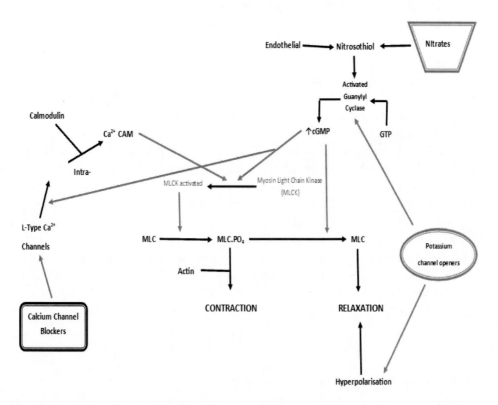

Figure 7. The mechanism of action of calcium channel blockers, potassium channel openers and nitrates (MLC, myosin light chain ; MLC.PO4,myosin light chain phosphate ; Ca2+, calcium ion; cGMP, cyclic guanosine monophosphate; GTP, guanosine triphosphate, CAM, calmodulin).

Pharmacokinetics

Most calcium channel blockers are well absorbed from the gastro-intestinal tract but undergo variable first passed metabolism. Verapamil and diltiazem have active, but less potent, metabolites.

The half-life of these agents range from 2 to 12 hours but modified release preparations can prolong their effect [8]. Amlodipine is more completely absorbed from the gastro-intestinal tract but its absorption is slow and it does not undergo first passed metabolism. It undergoes slower metabolism by the liver and therefore has a long duration of action which is approximately 36 hours [8].

Clinical Indication and Evidence Base

In the CAMELOT study [57] the effects of amlodipine were compared to placebo in patients with angina. Amlodipine was associated with a significant reduction in hospitalisation with angina and the need for revascularisation over a 2 year follow up period. Amlodipine was also compared to placebo in the CAPE study [58] with amlodipine showing significant reductions in the occurrence of ischaemia on Holter monitoring over a 7 week period.

Patients reported a reduction in the use of nitroglycerin (GTN) (67% versus 22%) and reduction in angina attacks (70% versus 44%) with amlodipine compared to placebo [58]. However, with the use of nifedipine, there was no reduction in primary endpoints (death, acute myocardial infarction, refractory angina, overt heart failure, debilitating stroke, and peripheral revascularisation) [59]. In the TIBET study [53], nifedipine was shown to reduce total ischaemic burden with an additive effect when combined with atenolol.

Side Effects

In the context of severely impaired left ventricular function, the reduced cardiac contractility associated with non-dihydropyridine calcium channel blockers, particularly verapamil, can result in the precipitation of acute heart failure with the development of pulmonary oedema and hypotension.

The negative chronotropic effect of these agents can also result in bradycardia, or the development of heart block. They should be used in caution in the context of pre-existing sinus bradycardia and atrio-ventricular node (AVN) disease or concomitant use of other rate limiting medications. They should not be used concomitantly with beta blockers as there is a risk of high grade atrio-ventricular node block. These agents can also alter gut motility and are very prone to causing constipation [8].

All calcium antagonists can result in arterial vasodilatation producing headache, dizziness and flushing but with continued use tolerance often occurs. An increase in trans-capillary hydrostatic pressure results in the development of ankle oedema which does not respond to diuretic therapy. Arterial vasodilatation is more of a problem with dihydropyridine calcium antagonists [8].

Potassium Channel Opener e.g. Nicorandil

Mechanism of Action

Nicorandil opens ATP sensitive channels resulting in hyper-polarisation in vascular smooth muscle cells inhibiting opening of L- type calcium channels resulting in systemic and coronary artery vasodilatation (figure 7). Nicorandil also carries a nitrate component which results in further vasodilatation through the generation of nitric oxide in vascular smooth muscle producing venodilatation (figure 6) [8].

Pharmacokinetics

Nicorandil is well absorbed from the gastrointestinal tract with the absorption being rapid. However, it has a short half-life of approximately one hour being eliminated by hepatic metabolism. The biological effects last up to 12 hours [8].

Clinical Indication and Evidence Base

In the IONA trial [60], nicorandil compared to placebo, when used as add on therapy to conventional drug treatment, showed a significant reduction in major coronary events. However, this was due to a reduction in 'hospital admission for cardiac chest pain' with no significant difference in non-fatal myocardial infarction and cardiac death [60].

Side Effects

Nicorandil can cause dizziness, nausea and vomiting [8]. Headache is common, being experienced by 25 to 50% of individuals, but continued use can result in tolerance [8]. Flushing and palpitations can also occur through reflex activation of the sympathetic nervous system [8].

Newer Anti-anginal Medication

Sinus Node Inhibitor e.g. Ivabradine

Mechanism of Action

Ivabradine acts by selectively inhibiting the cardiac pacemaker current If and has a negative chronotropic effect reducing heart rate both at rest and during exercise with effective anti-anginal properties [62-64]. If channels are highly expressed in the sino-atrial node and control mixed Na+–K+ inward current, If channels are activated by hyperpolarization and modulated by the autonomic nervous system (figure 8) [63, 64]. Inhibition is dose-dependent and baseline heart rate dependent with reductions in heart rate being greater in those with a higher baseline heart rate. Unlike beta blockers, ivabradine has no significant effect on cardiac contractility or blood pressure. Their effects are synergistic when combined with beta blockers with improved heart rate control and exercise capacity.

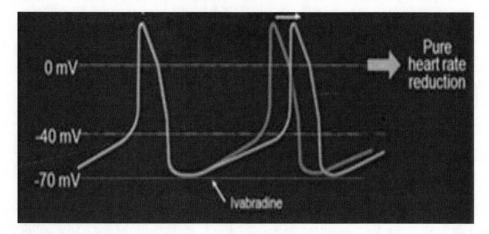

Figure 8. The effects of inhibiting the If channel resulting in reduction in heart rate through reducing the diastolic depolarisation slope in the sino-atrial node cells [65].

Pharmacokinetics

Ivabradine is well absorbed from the gastro-intestinal tract but undergoes first pass metabolism both in the wall of the gastro-intestinal tract and also the liver. It is metabolised through oxidation by the CYP3AIV enzyme but its metabolite remains active. The half-life of ivabradine is approximately 2 hours [8].

Clinical Indication and Evidence Base

Ivabradine is an effective agent when patients are intolerant to beta blockers or where the maximum tolerated dose of beta blockade has resulted in insufficient lowering of baseline heart rate. Bora et al. [66] showed ivabradine, when compared to placebo, resulted in improvements in exercise tolerance and time to development of myocardial ischaemia during exercise. When ivabradine was compared to atenolol, time to angina onset, number of angina attacks, use of short acting nitrates and total exercise duration were found to be similar in both groups [67]. Ivabradine was also found to be comparable to amlodipine with regards to total exercise duration, time to onset of angina, number of angina attacks and the consumption of short acting nitrates [68].

In the BEAUTIFUL study [69], in coronary heart disease patients with a heart rate more than 70 beats per minute, ivabradine significantly reduced the risk of coronary events by 22% (P=0.023), fatal and non-fatal myocardial infarction by 36% (P=0.001) and coronary revascularization by 30% (P=0.016).

Side Effects

Of patients taking ivabradine, 14.5% experience visual disturbance such as flashing lights and blurring of vision caused by inhibition of the Ih ion channels in the retina which are similar to the If receptor in the sino-atrial node [70]. This is experienced as a sensation of enhanced brightness in the context of maintained visual fields and acuity. The effect is mild, transient and fully reversible on cessation of ivabradine and lead to 1% of all patients in clinical trials to discontinue the use of the drug [70]. This sensation occurred on average 40 days after commencement of the ivabradine [70].

Bradycardia occurs at 2% and 5% for doses of 7.5 and 10 mg respectively (compared to 4.3% with atenolol) [70]. The use of ivabradine, or dose increments, should be avoided if the resting heart rate is less than 50 beats per minutes. First-degree AV block, ventricular extra systoles, dizziness and/or blurred vision occur in 1-10% of patients treated with ivabradine , with 2.6-4.8% reporting headache [70].

Late Sodium Current Inhibitor e.g. Ranolazine

Mechanism of Action

The mechanism of action of ranolazine is thought to be due to selective inhibition of late sodium influx across the sarcolemma and results in reductions in the abnormalities of ventricular repolarisation and contractility that accompany myocardial ischaemia (figure 9). There is only minimal reduction in systolic blood pressure and heart rate. Myocardial oxygen demand is reduced by reduced wall tension. Reduced wall tension also reduces compression of small intra-myocardial coronary vessels and result in improved myocardial perfusion.

Ranolazine, a partial fatty acid oxidation inhibitor, shifts ATP production from fatty acids to more oxygen efficient carbohydrate oxidation [71, 72].

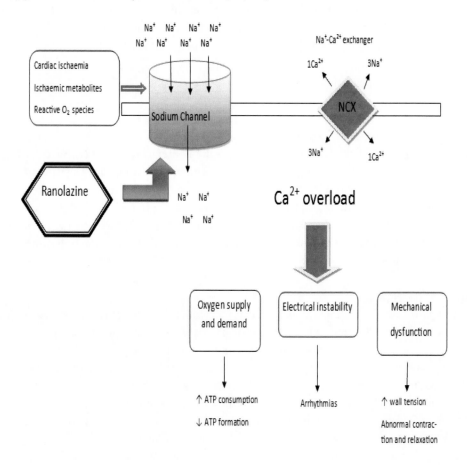

Figure 9. The mechanism of action of ranolazine with inhibition of late sodium influx, reducing the calcium overload which is detrimental to myocardial function.

Pharmacokinetics

Absorption from the gastrointestinal tract is only partial but ranolazine undergoes extensive metabolism through the CYP3A and CYP2D6 enzyme. It has a short half-life of approximately 2 hours which can be extended by modified release preparations [8].

Clinical Indication and Evidence Base

In the CARISA trial [73], ranolazine increased exercise capacity and provided additional anti-anginal relief in patients with symptomatic severe chronic angina taking standard doses of atenolol, amlodipine or diltiazem, without evident adverse, long-term survival consequences over 1 to 2 years of therapy. In the ERICA study [74], weekly consumption of long acting nitrates was reduced in patients who received a combination of amlodipine and ranolazine versus amlodipine alone.

Side Effects

Ranolazine can result in headache, dizziness and lethargy. Gastrointestinal symptoms such as nausea, dyspepsia and constipation can also occur. Cardiac arrhythmias can be precipitated through prolongation of the QTC interval and concomitant administration with other drugs that can prolong the QTC interval should be avoided [8].

Management in Special Groups

Cardiac Syndrome X

Cardiac Syndrome X is characterised by typical exercise induced angina, with a positive exercise stress ECG test or stress imaging, but in the context of normal coronary arteries on coronary angiography. The aetiology relates to abnormalities in the microcirculation during exertion. There is an abnormal dilator response in addition to an increased response to vasoconstrictors. Symptomatic benefit can be derived from nitrates [75], calcium antagonists [76] and beta blockers [77]. ACE inhibitors [78] and statins [79] are also beneficial in this condition, as is standard risk factor modification. Imipramine and aminophylline may be useful in providing symptomatic relief [80, 81].

Vasospastic Angina

Vasospastic angina patients experience typical angina symptoms, but these symptoms usually occur at rest and are caused by coronary artery spasm. Symptoms are particularly troublesome at night-time or during the early morning [82]. Coronary artery vasospasm and obstructive coronary artery disease are not mutually exclusive and patients may have a combination of both. The cause of vasospastic angina is thought to be due to hyper-reactivity of smooth muscle cells [83] in addition to endothelial dysfunction [84].

Treatment of vasospastic angina focuses on the use of nitrates and calcium antagonists to reduce vasospasm. High doses of calcium channel blockers may be required (480 mg per day of verapamil, 260 mg per day of diltiazem and 120 mg per day of nifedipine). In most patients, a combination of therapies may be useful in addition to combining dihydropyridine and non-dihydropyridine calcium blockers. Nicorandil may also be useful in patients who continue to have symptoms despite the use of nitrates and calcium antagonists [85]. If concomitant obstructive coronary artery disease is noted, in addition to suspected vasospasm, then standard prognosis modifying medication should be added.

Diabetic Patients

Management of symptomatic diabetic patients should mirror that of non-diabetics with risk factor modification, treatment of dyslipidaemia and hypertension. Good glycaemic control results in a substantial reduction in complications and mortality [86]. All patients should receive aspirin, a statin, ACE inhibitors and beta blockers to improve prognosis (assuming no contra-indications). ACE inhibitors reduce micro-albuminuria and the development of diabetic nephropathy. The aim should be to render the patient symptom free with a step-wise escalation in anti-anginal therapy. The management of silent ischemia is more difficult, with the use of 24 hour ambulatory ECG monitoring, it is estimated that up to two thirds of myocardial ischaemic episodes are silent [87-89]. In asymptomatic men between 40-59 years, the prevalence of silent ischaemia, as determined by coronary angiography, is

0.89% [88] with other studies suggesting a 1 -4% prevalence [91, 92]. This rises in asymptomatic diabetic individuals to 10-20% [93, 94], thus adding to the complexity of managing coronary artery disease in diabetics where the predominant symptom may be breathlessness. Beta blockers reduce the ischaemic load in silent ischaemia, prevent arrhythmias and cardiac remodelling, hence, improving outcome. The effect of atenolol 100mg, compared to placebo, was evaluated in the ASIST trial [93] with Holter monitoring. A reduction in ischaemic burden, prolonged event free survival and increased time to first event were noted [95]. Bisoprolol, in the TIBBS trial [96], resulted in a greater than 50% suppression of silent ischaemia with improved 1 year event free survival.

Female Patients

In the Euro Heart Survey of Stable Angina [97], female patients were shown to be less likely to have received effective secondary prevention. Female patients are also under-represented in clinical trials with limited female specific literature. However, their management should mirror those of male patients with effective secondary prevention and symptom control.

Hormone replacement therapy (HRT) with the combination of oral oestrogen and progesterone provides no cardiovascular benefit in women who have established coronary artery disease [98, 99]. However, there is an increased risk of developing cardiovascular disease in patients without established coronary artery disease. Therefore, HRT is not specifically recommended in patients with stable angina and current users should be advised to tapper doses towards discontinuation [100].

Elderly Patients

The potential physiological changes associated with advancing age develop at a different rate, and to a different extent, in each individual patient. Poly-pharmacy, increased risk of drug interaction, changes in bioavailability, elimination and increased sensitivity make the management of drug therapy in an elderly patient complex [97]. Increased side effects may reduce drug compliance [97]. Nonetheless, elderly patients should receive advice on risk factor modification, secondary prevention and symptom control with similar benefits seen from drug therapy, angioplasty and coronary bypass surgery compared to younger patients [102-104].

Conclusion

The medical management of stable angina is focused on improving prognosis by reducing progression to myocardial infarction and death. Antiplatelet drugs, statins, ACE inhibitors and beta blockers all have prognostic benefit. Secondly, the step-wise addition of anti-anginal therapy, starting with beta blockers, aims to minimise or abolish symptoms and improve quality of life. Each patient's medical treatment should be tailored to their characteristics and be an integral part of their general management including; patient education to promote motivation and compliance, risk factor modification, risk stratification and revascularisation with coronary angioplasty or bypass surgery.

References

[1]   Boden WE, O'Rourke RA, Teo KK, et al. Optimal medical therapy with or without PCI for stable coronary disease. *N Engl J Med* 2007; 356:1503-16.

[2]   Froehicher VF, Thompson AJ, Longo MR Jr et al. Value of exercise testing for screening asymptomatic men for latent coronary artery disease. *Prog Cardiovasc Dis* 1976;18:265-76.

[3]   Thaulow E, Erikssen J, Sandik L et al. Initial clinical presentation of cardiac disease in asymptomatic men with silent myocardial ischaemia and angiographically documented coronary artery disease: the Oslo ischemic study. *Am J Cardiol* 1993;72:629-33.

[4]   Langer A, Freeman MR, Josse RG, et al. Detection of silent myocardial ischaemia in diabetes mellitus. *Am J Cardiol* 1991;67:1073-8.

[5]   Naka M, Hiramatsu K, Aizawa T et al. Silent myocardial ischaemia in patients with non-insulin-dependent diabetes mellitus as judged by treadmill exercise testing and coronary angiography. *Am Heart J* 1992;123:46-53.

[6]   Fox K, Garcia MAA, Ardissino D et al. Guidelines on the management of angina pectoris. *European Heart Journal* 2006; 27:1341-1381.

[7]   Collaborative meta-analysis of randomised trials of anti-platelet therapy for prevention of death, myocardial infarction and stroke in high risk patients. *BMJ* 2002;324:71-86.

[8]   Waller DG, Renwick AG, Hillier K. *Medical Pharmacology and Therapeutics*, third edition. Saunders Elsevier. Chapter 5. 91-110.

[9]   Antithrombotic Trialists' Collaboration. Collaborative meta-analysis of randomised trials of antiplatelet therapy for prevention of death, myocardial infarction, and stroke in high risk patients. *BMJ* 2002;324:71–86.

[10]   Juul-Moller S, Edvardsson N, Jahnmatz B et al. Double-blind trial of aspirin in primary prevention of myocardial infarction in patients with stable chronic angina pectoris. The Swedish Angina Pectoris Aspirin Trial (SAPAT) Group. *Lancet* 1992;340:1421–1425.

[11]   Patrono C, Coller B, FitzGerald GA et al. Platelet-active drugs: the relationships among dose, effectiveness, and side effects: the Seventh ACCP Conference on Antithrombotic and Thrombolytic Therapy. *Chest* 2004;126(Suppl. 3):234S–264S.

[12]   Weil J, Colin-Jones D, Langman M et al. Prophylactic aspirin and risk of peptic ulcer bleeding. *BMJ* 1995;310:827–830.

[13]   Derry S, Loke YK. Risk of gastrointestinal haemorrhage with long term use of aspirin: meta-analysis. *BMJ* 2000;321:1183–1187.

[14]   Chan FK, Ching JY, Hung LC et al. Clopidogrel versus aspirin and esomeprazole to prevent recurrent ulcer bleeding. *N Engl J Med* 2005; 352:238–244.

[15]   Sudlow C, Baigent C. The adverse effects of different doses of aspirin: a systematic review of randomised trials and observational studies. (Abstract). *Stroke* 2000; 31:2869.

[16]   Antiplatelet Trialists' Collaboration. Collaborative overview of randomised trials of antiplatelet therapy–I: Prevention of death, myocardial infarction, and stroke by prolonged antiplatelet therapy in various categories of patients. *BMJ* 1994; 308:81–106.

[17]   McKee SA, Sane DC, Deliargyris EN. Aspirin resistance in cardiovascular disease: a review of prevalence, mechanisms, and clinical significance. *Thromb Haemost.* 2002;88: 711–715.

[18] Eikelboom JW, Hirsh J, Weitz JI, et al. Aspirin-resistant thromboxane biosynthesis and the risk of myocardial infarction, stroke, or cardiovascular death in patients at high risk for cardiovascular events. *Circulation.* 2002; 105: 1650–1655.

[19] von Beckerath N, Taubert D, Pogatsa-Murray G, Schomig E, Kastrati A, Schomig A. Absorption, metabolization, and antiplatelet effects of 300-, 600-, and 900-mg loading doses of clopidogrel: results of the ISAR-CHOICE (Intracoronary Stenting and Antithrombotic Regimen: Choose Between 3 High Oral Doses for Immediate Clopidogrel Effect) Trial. *Circulation.* 2005; 112: 2946–2950.

[20] CAPRIE Steering Committee. A randomised, blinded, trial of clopidogrel versus aspirin in patients at risk of ischaemic events (CAPRIE). *Lancet* 1996; 348:1329–1339.

[21] Bhatt DL, Fox KAA, Hacke W et al for the CHARISMA Investigators. Clopidogrel and Aspirin versus Aspirin Alone for the Prevention of Atherothrombotic Events. *N Engl J Med* 2006; 354:1706-1717April 20, 2006.

[22] The Clopidogrel in Unstable Angina to Prevent Recurrent Events (CURE) trial investigators. effects of clopidogrel in addition to aspirin in patients with acute coronary syndromes without ST-segment elevation. *N Engl J Med* 2001; 345:494-502.

[23] Gurbel PA, Bliden KP, Hiatt BL, et al. Clopidogrel for coronary stenting: response variability, drug resistance, and the effect of pretreatment platelet reactivity. *Circulation.* 2003;107: 2908–2913.

[24] Muller I, Besta F, Schulz C, et al. Prevalence of clopidogrel non-responders among patients with stable angina pectoris scheduled for elective coronary stent placement. *Thromb Haemost.* 2003;89: 783–787.

[25] Jaremo P, Lindahl TL, Fransson SG, et al. Individual variations of platelet inhibition after loading doses of clopidogrel. *J Intern Med.* 2002;252: 233–238.

[26] Gurbel PA, Bliden KP. Durability of platelet inhibition by clopidogrel. *Am J Cardiol.* 2003;91: 1123–1125.

[27] Matetzky S, Shenkman B, Guetta V, et al. Clopidogrel resistance is associated with increased risk of recurrent atherothrombotic events in patients with acute myocardial infarction. *Circulation.* 2004;109: 3171–3175.

[28] Lau WC, Gurbel PA, Watkins PB, et al. Contribution of hepatic cytochrome P450 3A4 metabolic activity to the phenomenon of clopidogrel resistance. *Circulation.* 2004;109: 166–171.

[29] Kaufmann PA, Mandinov L, Seiler C et al. Impact of exercise-induced coronary vasomotion on anti-ischaemic therapy. *Coron Artery Dis* 2000;11:363–369.

[30] Grundy SM, Cleeman JI, Merz CN et al. Implications of recent clinical trials for the National Cholesterol Education Program Adult Treatment Panel III Guidelines. *J Am Coll Cardiol* 2004; 44:720–732.

[31] Randomised trila of cholesterol lowering in 4444 patients with coronary artery disease: the Scandinavian Simvastatin Survival Study (4S). *Lancet* 1994; 344:1383-9.

[32] MRC/BHF Heart protection Study of cholesterol lowering with simvastatin in 20,536 high risk individuals: a randomised placebo controlled trial. *Lancet* 2002; 360:7-22.

[33] Sacks FM, Tomkin AM, Shepherd J, et al. effects of pravastatin on coronary disease events in subgroups defined by coronary risk factors: the Prospective Pravastatin Pooling Project. *Circulation 2000;* 102:1893-900.

[34] JBS 2: Joint British Societies' guidelines on prevention of cardiovascular disease in clinical practice. *Heart*2005; 91.

[35] Faggiotto A, Paoletti R. State-of-the-Art lecture. Statins and blockers of the renin-angiotensin system: vascular protection beyond their primary mode of action. *Hypertension* 1999; 34:987–996.

[36] Ridker PM, Cannon CP, Morrow D et al. C-reactive protein levels and outcomes after statin therapy. *N Engl J Med* 2005; 352:20–28.

[37] Pasceri V, Patti G, Nusca A et al. Randomized trial of atorvastatin for reduction of myocardial damage during coronary intervention: results from the ARMYDA (Atorvastatin for Reduction of MYocardial Damage during Angioplasty) study. *Circulation* 2004; 110:674–678.

[38] Keech A, Simes RJ, Barter P et al FIELD study investigators. Effects of long-term fenofibrate therapy on cardiovascular events in 9795 people with type 2 diabetes mellitus (the FIELD study): randomised controlled trial. *Lancet* 2005; 366:1829–1831.

[39] Studer M, Briel M, Leimenstoll B et al. Effect of different anti-lipidemic agents and diets on mortality: a systematic review. *Arch Intern Med* 2005; 165:725–730.

[40] LaRosa JC, Grundy SM, Waters DD et al. Intensive lipid lowering with atorvastatin in patients with stable coronary disease. *N Engl J Med* 2005; 352:1425–1435.

[41] Pedersen TR, Faergeman O, Kastelein JJ et al. High-dose atorvastatin versus usual-dose simvastatin for secondary prevention after myocardial infarction: the IDEAL study: a randomized controlled trial. *JAMA* 2005; 294:2437–2445.

[42] Prueksaritanont T, Tang C, Qiu Y et al. Effects of fibrates on metabolism of statins in human hepatocytes. *Drug Metab Dispos* 2002; 30:1280–1287.

[43] Fox KM. Efficacy of perindopril in reduction of cardiovascular events among patients with stable coronary artery disease: randomised, double-blind, placebo-controlled, multicenter trial (the EUROPA study). *Lancet* 2003; 362: 782-8.

[44] Yusuf S, Sleight P, Bosch J et al. Effects of angiotensin-converting-enzyme inhibitor, ramipril, on cardiovascular events in high-risk patients. The Heart Outcomes Prevention Evaluation Study Investigators. *N Engl J Med* 2000; 342: 145-53.

[45] Pfeffer MA, McMurray JJ, Velazquez EJ et al. Valsartan, captopril, or both in myocardial infarction complicated by heart failure, left ventricular dysfunction, or both. *N Engl J Med* 2003; 349:1893–1906.

[46] Yusuf S, Pfeffer MA, Swedberg K et al. Effects of candesartan in patients with chronic heart failure and preserved left-ventricular ejection fraction: the CHARM-Preserved Trial. *Lancet* 2003; 362:777–781.

[47] Rose GA, Blackburn H. Cardiovascular survey methods. *Monogr Ser World Health Organ* 1968;56:1–188.

[48] Cook DG, Shaper AG, MacFarlane PW. Using the WHO (Rose) angina questionnaire in cardiovascular epidemiology. *Int J Epidemiol* 1989;18: 607–613.

[49] Effect of metoprolol CR/XL in chronic heart failure: Metoprolol CR/XL *Randomized Intervention Trial in Congestive Heart* Failure (MERIT-HF). Lancet 1999; 353:2001–2007.

[50] The Cardiac Insufficiency Bisoprolol Study II (CIBIS-II): a randomized trial. *Lancet* 1999; 353:9–13.

[51] Poole-Wilson PA, Swedberg K, Cleland JG et al. Comparison of carvedilol and metoprolol on clinical outcomes in patients with chronic heart failure in the Carvedilol Or Metoprolol European Trial (COMET): randomized controlled trial. *Lancet*. 2003 Jul 5; 362(9377):7-13.

[52] Rehnqvist N, Hjemdahl P, Billing E et al. Effects of metoprolol vs. verapamil in patients with stable angina pectoris. The Angina Prognosis Study in Stockholm (APSIS). *Eur Heart J* 1996; 17:76–81.

[53] Dargie HJ, Ford I, Fox KM. Total Ischaemic Burden European Trial (TIBET). Effects of ischaemia and treatment with atenolol, nifedipine SR and their combination on outcome in patients with chronic stable angina. The TIBET Study Group. *Eur Heart J* 1996; 17:104–112.

[54] Pepine CJ, Cohn PF, Deedwania PC et al. Effects of treatment on outcome in mildly symptomatic patients with ischaemia during daily life. The Atenolol Silent Ischemia Study (ASIST). *Circulation* 1994; 90:762–768.

[55] Gibbons RJ, Chatterjee K, Daley J et al. ACC/AHA/ACP-ASIM guidelines for the management of patients with chronic stable angina: a report of the American College of Cardiology/American Heart Association Task Force on Practice Guidelines (Committee on Management of Patients With Chronic Stable Angina). *J Am Coll Cardiol* 1999; 33:2092–2197.

[56] ISIS-4 (Fourth International Study of Infarct Survival) Collaborative Group. ISIS-4: a randomized factorial trial assessing early oral captopril, oral mononitrate, and intravenous magnesium sulphate in 58,050 patients with suspected acute myocardial infarction. *Lancet* 1995; 345:669–685.

[57] Nissen SE, Tuzcu EM, Libby P et al. Effect of antihypertensive agents on cardio-vascular events in patients with coronary disease and normal blood pressure: the CAMELOT study: a randomized controlled trial. *JAMA* 2004; 292:2217–2225.

[58] Deanfield JE, Detry JM, Lichtlen PR et al. Amlodipine reduces transient myocardial ischemia in patients with coronary artery disease: double-blind Circadian Anti-Ischemia Program in Europe (CAPE Trial). *J Am Coll Cardiol* 1994; 24:1460–1467.

[59] Poole-Wilson PA, Lubsen J, Kirwan BA et al. Effect of long-acting nifedipine on mortality and cardiovascular morbidity in patients with stable angina requiring treatment (ACTION trial): randomized controlled trial. *Lancet* 2004; 364:849–857.

[60] Effect of nicorandil on coronary events in patients with stable angina: the Impact Of Nicorandil in Angina (IONA) randomized trial. *Lancet* 2002; 359:1269–1275.

[61] Fox KM. Efficacy of perindopril in reduction of cardiovascular events among patients with stable coronary artery disease: randomized, double-blind, placebo-controlled, multicentre trial (the EUROPA study). *Lancet* 2003; 362:782–788.

[62] Tardif JC, Ford I, Tendera M et al. Efficacy of ivabradine, a new selective If inhibitor, compared with atenolol in patients with chronic stable angina. *Eur Heart J* 2005; 26:2529–2536.

[63] Thollon C, Cambarrat C, Vian J et al. Electrophysiological effects of S 16257, a novel sino-atrial node modulator, on rabbit and guinea-pig cardiac preparations: comparison with UL-FS 49. *Br. J. Pharmacol* 1994. 112 (1): 37–42.

[64] Sulfi S, Timmis AD (2006). "Ivabradine – the first selective sinus node If channel inhibitor in the treatment of stable angina". *Int. J. Clin. Pract.* 60 (2): 222–8.

[65] Borer JS, Fox K, Jaillon P et al. Anti-anginal and anti-ischemic effects of ivabradine, an I(f) inhibitor, in stable angina: a randomized, double-blind, multicenter, placebo-controlled trial. *Circulation* 2003; 107:817–823.

[66] Borer JS, Ford I, Jaillon P et al. Anti-anginal and anti-ischaemic effects of ivabradine, an If inhibitor, in stable angina: A randomized, double-blind, multicenter, placebo-controlled trial. *Circulation* 2003; 107:817-23.

[67] Tardif JC, Ford I, Tendera M et al, Efficacy of ivabradine, a new selective If inhibitor, compared with atenolol in patients in chronic stable angina. *Eur Heart J* 2005; 26:2529-36.

[68] Ruzyllo W, Tendera M, Ford I et al. Anti-anginal efficacy and safety of ivabradine, compared with amlodipine, in patients with stable effort angina pectoris: a three month, randomized, double-blind, multi-center, non-inferiority trial. *Drugs* 2007; 67:393-405.

[69] Fox K, Ford I, Steg PG et al. Ivabradine for patients with stable coronary artery disease and left-ventricular systolic dysfunction: a randomized, double-blind, placebo-controlled trial. *The Lancet* 2008;372 (9641): 807–816.

[70] Tardif JC, Ford I, Tendera M et al. Efficacy of ivabradine, a new selective I(f) inhibitor, compared with atenolol in patients with chronic stable angina. *Eur. Heart J* 2005. 26 (23): 2529–36.

[71] *Ranolazine: A novel partial inhibitor of fatty acid oxidation for angina;* KN Mahesh Kumar, S Sandhiya; Department of Pharmacology, Jawaharlal Institute of Postgraduate Medical Education and Research (JIPMER), Pondicherry - 605 006, India; http://www.ijp-online.com/ article.asp?issn=0253-7613;year=2006; volume=38;issue=4; spage=302;epage=304;aulast=Mahesh

[72] European Journal of Heart Failure; Partial fatty acid oxidation inhibitors: a potentially new class of drugs for heart failure; http://eurjhf.oxfordjournals.org/ content/4/1/3. full.pdf+html

[73] Chaitman BR, Pepine CJ, Parker JO et al for the Combination Assessment of Ranolazine In Stable Angina (CARISA) Investigators. Effects of ranolazine with atenolol, amlodipine, or diltiazem on exercise tolerance and angina frequency in patients with severe chronic angina. A randomized controlled trial. *JAMA* 2004;291:309–16.

[74] Stone PH, Gratsiansky NA, Blokhin A et al. Anti-anginal efficacy of ranolazine when added to treatment with amlodipine. The ERICA trail. *J Am Coll Cardiol* 2006; 38:566-75.

[75] Kaski JC, Rosano GM, Collins P et al. Cardiac syndrome X: clinical characteristics and left ventricular function. Long-term follow-up study. *J Am Coll Cardiol* 1995; 25:807–814.

[76] Cannon RO III, Watson RM, Rosing DR et al. Efficacy of calcium channel blocker therapy for angina pectoris resulting from small-vessel coronary artery disease and abnormal vasodilator reserve. *Am J Cardiol* 1985; 56:242–246.

[77] Lanza GA, Colonna G, Pasceri V et al. Atenolol versus amlodipine versus isosorbide-5-mononitrate on anginal symptoms in syndrome X. *Am J Cardiol* 1999;84:854–856. A8.

[78] Ozcelik F, Altun A, Ozbay G. Anti-anginal and anti-ischaemic effects of nisoldipine and ramipril in patients with syndrome X. *Clin Cardiol* 1999; 22:361–365.

[79] Kayikcioglu M, Payzin S, Yavuzgil O et al. Benefits of statin treatment in cardiac syndrome-X1. *Eur Heart J* 2003; 24:1999–2005.

[80] Cannon RO III, Quyyumi AA, Mincemoyer R et al. Imipramine in patients with chest pain despite normal coronary angiograms. *N Engl J Med* 1994; 330:1411–1417.

[81] Yoshio H, Shimizu M, Kita Y et al. Effects of short-term aminophylline administration on cardiac functional reserve in patients with syndrome X. *J Am Coll Cardiol* 1995; 25:1547–1551.

[82] Hillis LD, Braunwald E. Coronary-artery spasm. *N Engl J Med* 1978; 299:695–702.

[83] Kaski JC, Crea F, Meran D et al. Local coronary supersensitivity to diverse vasoconstrictive stimuli in patients with variant angina. *Circulation* 1986;74:1255–1265.

[84] Nakayama M, Yasue H, Yoshimura M et al. T-786–.C mutation in the 5'-flanking region of the endothelial nitric oxide synthase gene is associated with coronary spasm. *Circulation* 1999; 99:2864–2870.

[85] Lablanche JM, Bauters C, McFadden EP, Quandalle P, Bertrand ME. Potassium channel activators in vasospastic angina. *Eur Heart J* 1993;14(Suppl. B):22–24.

[86] UK Prospective Diabetes Study (UKPDS) Group. Intensive blood glucose control with sulphonyureas or insulin compared with conventional treatment and risk of complications in patients with Type 2 diabetes (UKPDS 33). *Lancet* 1998; 352:837–53.

[87] Deedwania PC, Carbajal EV. Silent myocardial ischaemia: a clinical perspective. *Arch Intern Med* 1991; 151:2373-82.

[88] L angou RA, Huang EK, Kelley MK et al. Predictive accuracy of coronary artery calcification and abnormal exercise test for coronary artery disease in asymptomatic men. *Circulation* 1980; 62:1196-203.

[89] Yeung AC, Barry J, Orav J et al. Effect of asymptomatic ischaemia on long-term prognosis in chronic stable coronary disease. *Circulation* 1991; 83:1598-604.

[90] Fazzini PF, Prati PL, Rovelli F et al. Epidemiology of silent myocardial ischaemia in asymptomatic middle-aged men (the ECCIS Project). *Am J Cardiol* 1993; 72:1383-8.

[91] Froehicher VF, Thompson AJ, Longo MR Jr et al. Value of exercise testing for screening asymptomatic men for latent coronary artery disease. *Prog Cardiovasc Dis* 1976; 18:265-76.

[92] Thaulow E, Erikssen J, Sandik L et al. Initial clinical presentation of cardiac disease in asymptomatic men with silent myocardial ischaemia and angiographically documented coronary artery disease: the Oslo ischemic study. *Am J Cardiol* 1993; 72:629-33.

[93] Langer A, Freeman MR, Josse RG, et al. Detection of silent myocardial ischaemia in diabetes mellitus. *Am J Cardiol* 1991; 67:1073-8.

[94] Naka M, Hiramatsu K, Aizawa T et al. Silent myocardial ischaemia in patients with non-insulin-dependent diabetes mellitus as judged by treadmill exercise testing and coronary angiography. *Am Heart J* 1992; 123:46-53.

[95] Pepine CJ, Cohn PF, Deedwania PC et al. Effects of treatment on outcome in mildly symptomatic patients with ischaemia during daily life. The Atenolol Silent Ischaemia Study. *Circulation* 1994:90; 762-8.

[96] Von Arnim T. The TIBBS Investigators. Prognostic significance of transient ischemic episodes: Response to treatment shows improved prognosis. Results of the Total Ischemic Burden Bisoprolol Study (TIBBS) Follow-up. *J Am Coll Cardiol* 1996; 28:20-4.

[97] Daly CA, Clemens F, Sendon JL et al. Euro Heart Survey Investigators. Gender differences in the management and clinical outcome of stable angina. *Circulation* 2006; 113:467–469.

[98]   Hulley S, Grady D, Bush T et al. Randomized trial of estrogen plus progestin for secondary prevention of coronary heart disease in postmenopausal women. Heart and Estrogen/progestin Replacement Study (HERS) Research Group. *JAMA* 1998; 280:605–613.

[99]   Grady D, Herrington D, Bittner V et al. Cardiovascular disease outcomes during 6.8 years of hormone therapy: Heart and Estrogen/progestin Replacement Study follow-up (HERS II). *JAMA* 2002;288:49–57.

[100] Hersh AL, Stefanick ML, Stafford RS. National use of postmenopausal hormone therapy: annual trends and response to recent evidence. *JAMA* 2004;291:47–53.

[101] Montamat SC, Cusack BJ, Vestal RE. Management of drug therapy in the elderly. *N Engl J Med* 1989;321:303–309.

[102] Gundersen T, Abrahamsen AM, Kjekshus J et al. Timolol-related reduction in mortality and reinfarction in patients ages 65-75 years surviving acute myocardial infarction. Prepared for the Norwegian Multicentre Study Group. *Circulation* 1982;66:1179–1184.

[103] Metzger JP, Tabone X, Georges JL et al. Coronary angioplasty in patients 75 years and older; comparison with coronary bypass surgery. *Eur Heart J* 1994;15:213–217.

[104] Bonnier H, de Vries C, Michels R et al. Initial and long-term results of coronary angioplasty and coronary bypass surgery in patients of 75 or older. *Br Heart J* 1993;70:122–125.

In: Current Issues in the Management of Stable Ischemic Heart …   ISBN: 978-1-62417-203-8
Editor: Mukesh Singh   © 2013 Nova Science Publishers, Inc.

Chapter V

Chronic Stable Angina: Treatment Modalities Beyond the Guidelines

Beevash Ray[*] *and Kevin Marzo*

Winthrop University Hospital, Mineola, New York, US

Abstract

Although improvements over the last 40 years have occurred, death from ischemic cardiac diseases remains the number one killer of adults. Chronic stable angina is the presenting symptom of ischemic cardiac disease in a majority of patients. However, strategies for the treatment of chronic stable angina remain controversial and fairly dynamic. Guidelines, originally written a decade ago, suggest optimal medical therapy (OMT) and revascularization as the cornerstones of treatment. Yet, recent studies such as BARI-2 and COURAGE have put into question the utility of revascularization and the definition of OMT has become blurred. In this review we will examine the role of revascularization, and investigate new pharmacological agents for the treatment of chronic stable angina. Furthermore, novel treatments such spinal cord stimulation (SCS), enhanced external counter compulsion (EECP), and transmyocardial laser revascularization (TMLR) will also be explored.

Introduction

Over the last 40 years, great strides have been made in reducing death from cardiovascular diseases. However, coronary artery disease (CAD) remains a significant source of morbidity and mortality in the United States, as well as the world. It is estimated

---
[*] Address for correspondence: Beevash Ray, MD, 120 Mineola Blvd., Suite 500, Mineola, NY 11501. (516) 663 – 4480.

that 13,200,000 Americans have CAD, 6,500,000 of whom have angina pectoris with 400,000 new cases yearly. [1] From an economic standpoint the costs are staggering. In 2010, the estimated direct and indirect cost of CAD was $177.1 billion. [2] Furthermore, $11.7 billion was paid to Medicare beneficiaries for in-hospital costs in 2006 when CHD was the principal diagnosis ($14,009 per discharge for AMI, $12,977 per discharge for coronary atherosclerosis, and $10,630 per discharge for other ischemic HD). [3] Finally, disability related to CAD is projected to increase to over 80 million disability-adjusted life-years globally by 2020. [4]

Management paradigms for treating angina revolve around reducing symptoms related to ischemia and preventing myocardial infarction or sudden cardiac death. Traditional options for CAD treatment include medical therapy and coronary revascularization. Background medical therapy is recommended for all stages of CAD. The benefits of coronary revascularization have been well established in the context of acute coronary syndromes (ACS) with ST-segment elevations and non-ST-segment elevation myocardial infarction (MI). [5] Unfortunately, the guidelines for chronic stable angina by the major cardiology societies such the American College of Cardiology (ACC) and American Heart Association (AHA) were established in 2002 and most recently updated in 2007. However, since then the role of revascularization in CAD has been evolving in patients with chronic stable angina. Furthermore, novel treatments of angina such as spinal cord stimulation (SCS), enhanced external counter compulsion (EECP), and transmyocardial laser revascularization (TMLR) as well as newer pharmacologic agents may also provide symptomatic relief for refractory angina.

Angina

The classical description of angina pectoris is a clinical syndrome that consists of discomfort or pain in the chest, jaw, shoulder, back, or arm. It is usually graded as typical, atypical, and non-cardiac based on the qualities of the symptoms. [6] Angina can also be categorized by using the Canadian Cardiovascular Society Functional Classification of Angina Pectoris. [7] From a pathophysiology standpoint, it is felt that angina reflects inadequate oxygen supply for myocardial metabolic demands with resultant ischemia. This condition is usually a result of atherosclerotic disease of the coronary arteries, causing a critical narrowing of the vessels, thus reducing the oxygen supply of the myocardium. Other variables that affect this mismatch include heart rate, contractility, and wall tension, which can be deeply affected by the patient's systolic pressures and overall volume state.

Treatment Overview

Medications

The goal of treatment is to reduce and or eliminate the above mismatch of oxygen demand versus oxygen supply. This has traditionally been achieved by using medication and/or revascularization techniques. Over the years several pharmacological agents have been approved for treatment of CAD. They include nitrates, beta-adrenergic blockers, calcium channel blockers, statins, anti-platelet agents, and angiotensin-converting enzyme inhibitors (ACE-I)/angiotensin receptor blockers (ARB's). [8] The combination of these medications with dose modifications based on LDL and dose maximization limited by blood pressure and heart rare comprise optimal medical management (OMT). Evidence for the efficacy of these medications can be found throughout the angina literature and in various guidelines. [9] This is also the regimen that has been used in studies such as Clinical Outcomes Utilizing Revascularization and Aggressive Drug Evaluation (COURAGE) when evaluating OMT versus percutaneous intervention.

Interventional Therapy

Interventional therapy for angina can be separated into two categories, coronary artery bypass surgery (CABG) and percutaneous intervention (PCI). CABG has an over 30 year history of success for the treatment of CAD. It is an open surgical procedure which involves the use of autologous arteries or veins to reroute blood around relatively stenotic segments of the proximal coronary artery thereby increasing blood flow to ischemic areas. Data from the 1970s showed occlusion rates of saphenous vein grafts of 10% to 15% within one week to one year after operation and 20% to 25% by five years after surgery. [10] The use of internal mammary arteries have better data as more than 90% of grafts are still functioning more than 10 years after surgery. CABG has consistently been shown to improve the symptoms of patients with angina. Observational studies have noted freedom from angina for approximately 80% of patients at five years post operation. [11]

PCI originally began as percutaneous transcatheter angioplasty (PTCA) in 1977 with catheter based balloon inflation of stenotic areas of the coronary arteries. However, restenosis rates were high early on for these balloon-only techniques, occurring in approximately 30 to 50 percent of patients. [12] This procedure later evolved with the incorporation of mechanical debulking devices as well as stents, both drug eluting (DES) and bare metal (BMS). Subsequently, restenosis rates have dropped by over 30%. [13] There are several advantages of using PCI for the treatment of CAD over CABG including a low level of procedure-related morbidity and mortality, a shorter hospital stay, an earlier return to activity, and the feasibility of multiple procedures. The disadvantages of PCI are that it is not feasible in all patients, its significant incidence of restenosis, and the occasional need for emergency CABG surgery. However, these issues are becoming less important as newer technologies have made the procedure both safer and reduced restenosis rates.

Medical Therapy versus Revascularization

There have been more than 30 randomized trials comparing medical therapy to revascularization strategies for the management of angina. [14] However, varying type of revascularization techniques were used in these trials as well as differing definitions of optimal medical therapy. Of the trials mentioned, 13 of them were CABG only with 6 of them those using saphenous vein grafts only. Furthermore in the contemporary trials only one used significant numbers of DES. Because most of these trials do not reflect the current standard of care of medications and revascularization techniques, only two of the more contemporary trials will be reviewed here, Bypass and Revascularization Investigation 2 Diabetes (BARI-2D) and Clinical Outcomes Utilizing Aggressive Drug Evaluation (COURAGE). [15]

COURAGE compared myocardial revascularization plus optimal medical therapy versus optimal medical therapy alone in 2,287 randomized patients. Patients eligible for enrollment were those with chronic angina (CCS) Class I–III, stable post-MI patients, and asymptomatic patients with objective evidence of myocardial ischemia. About half of the patients had minimal or no symptoms of angina and the extent of ischemia as assessed by nuclear imaging prior to treatment in a subset of patients were not severe. The primary outcome of the trial was death from any cause and nonfatal myocardial infarction during a follow-up period of 2.5 to 7.0 years (median, 4.6). There were 211 primary events in the PCI group (19%) and 202 events in the medical therapy group (18.5%) with the hazard ratio for the PCI group, 1.05; 95% confidence interval [CI], 0.87 to 1.27; P = 0.62. Thus, the authors concluded as an initial management strategy in patients with stable coronary artery disease, PCI did not reduce the risk of death, myocardial infarction, or other major cardiovascular events when added to optimal medical therapy. In terms of angina relief, there was a statistically significant difference in the rates of freedom from angina throughout most of the follow-up period, in favor of the PCI group. But at 5 years, 74% of patients in the PCI group and 72% of those in the medical therapy group were free of angina (P = 0.35). [16]

The BARI 2D trial investigated whether revascularization with PCI or CABG would confer additional benefit to intensive medical therapy in patients with diabetes and CAD. There were 2,368 patients randomized to the 2 cohorts and the primary endpoints included death and a composite of death, myocardial infarction, or stroke (major cardiovascular events). Patients were excluded if they had left main disease or needed urgent revascu-larization, had a revascularization procedure in the previous 6 months, or other major comorbidities. At 5 years, rates of survival did not differ significantly between the revascularization group (88.3%) and the medical-therapy group (87.8%, P = 0.97). Interestingly, at 5 years, 42.1% of the patients in the medical therapy group had undergone clinically indicated revascularization, with almost half of these procedures occurring within the first year and 11% of these events precipitated by an MI. Furthermore, the use of DES (35%) was low as was the use of thienopyridines (21%). Unlike COURAGE, angina relief was not investigated in this trial. [17]

Although BARI 2D and COURAGE are the two most current randomized trials that can be found in the literature, neither trial is a true reflection of revascularization techniques and medical therapies used today. The lack of DES use as well as newer anti-angina medical therapies such as ranolazine put into question the utility of these studies in the modern era. Based on these studies we can only conclude there is no mortality benefit to revascularization on those previous treatment strategies, yet there is significant angina relief early on with revascularization. Newer studies are being planned to both incorporate newer technologies and select specific populations that may benefit most from one or the other treatment strategy. One such study is The International Study of Comparative Health Effectiveness with Medical and Invasive Approaches (ISCHEMIA) which will compare angiography and revascularization plus optimal medical therapy with the conservative strategy of optimal medical therapy only using stress test and CT angiography directed care. ISCHEMIA's primary end point is time to cardiovascular death, MI, or hospitalization for unstable angina, resuscitated cardiac arrest, or heart failure and the secondary end points include angina-related quality of life and cost-effectiveness. [17] Another study, the Fractional Flow Reserve (FFR) Guided Percutaneous Coronary Intervention Plus OMT Verses OMT (FAME II) trial will hopefully shed more light on whether populations with FFR guided treatment have better outcomes than OMT only. [18]

Alternative Angina Therapies

Patients who are on OMT, ineligible for revascularization, and still have angina are deemed to have refractory angina. The ECS actually defined refractory angina has having four distinct qualities: (1) angina caused by coronary insufficiency;(2) cannot be controlled by a combination of medical therapy, angioplasty and coronary bypass surgery;(3) reversible myocardial ischemia should be clinically established; and (4) occurring for a duration of more than 3 months. [19] For these patients alternative treatment strategies have been proposed. The ACC/AHA Guidelines on Chronic Stable Angina list 3 such strategies: Spinal Cord Stimulation (SCS), Enhanced External Counter Compulsion (EECP), and Transmyocardial Laser Revascularization (TMLR). These strategies have received either class IIA (TMLR) or IIB (EECP and SCS) recommendations. However, no updates have been made to these recommendations since 2002. Furthermore, a newer anti-angina medication, ranolazine was only mentioned once in those guidelines with no actual class recommendations. [20]

Ranolazine

Ranolazine was approved by the FDA for treatment of chronic angina in 2006 and is a novel anti-angina agent. Unlike other anti-angina agents, it does work not through an effect on heart rate, the hemodynamic state, the inotropic state, or an increase in coronary blood flow. The exact mechanism by which it works is still unclear. It was initially thought to act via its property as a partial fatty acid oxide inhibitor, which shifts ATP production from fatty acids to more oxygen efficient carbohydrate oxidation. These pharmacological effects, however, were generally observed at concentrations in excess of therapeutic plasma concentrations in human clinical trials (10 mol/L). [21] More recent evidence suggests that ranolazine reduces calcium overload in the ischemic myocyte through inhibition of the late sodium current. [22]

There have been four randomized, double-blind trials that have demonstrated that ranolazine reduces frequency of angina episodes and nitroglycerin consumption and improves exercise duration and time to angina attacks. [23] The Combination Assessment of Ranolazine and Stable Angina (CARISA) trial was a blinded randomized control trial (RCT) in which 823 adults with symptomatic chronic angina on at least one antianginal were assigned to receive placebo, 750mg, or 1000mg of twice daily ranolazine. [24] The endpoints investigated were change in exercise duration, time to onset of angina, time to onset of ischemia, nitroglycerin use, and number of angina attacks. Trough exercise duration increased by 115.6 seconds from baseline in both ranolazine groups (pooled) vs. 91.7 seconds in the placebo group ($P = .01$) and reduced angina attacks and nitroglycerin use by about 1 per week vs. placebo ($P<.02$). In a follow-up RCT, MERLIN TIMI 36, ranolazine was used in an

ACS population to determine if there was any benefit in the composite primary endpoint of cardiovascular death, myocardial infarction (MI), or recurrent ischemia. Although there was no benefit in the primary endpoint, the study did show there was significant benefit in angina relief. Consequently, ranolazine is an effective medication for symptomatic angina relief but does not provide any mortality benefit. [25]

Enhanced External Counterpulsation (EECP)

As early as 1953, scientists have been working on counterpulsation, showing that this technique markedly reduces the workload, and thus oxygen consumption, of the left ventricle. [26] EECP therapy consists of electrocardiogram-gated sequential compression of the lower extremities occurring during diastole, followed by simultaneous decompression during systole. These compressions increase venous return, decrease left ventricular afterload and increase diastolic filling pressure in the coronary arteries. Mechanistically, it is similar to the intra-aortic balloon pump in increasing coronary flow and decreasing afterload. The typical course of treatment consists of thirty-five 1-hour sessions over a period of 7 weeks.

Recently the Cochrane Group did a review of all EECP papers to determine the efficacy of this technique. Over 300 studies were investigated and only one met the criteria of a being a RCT of EECP vs. sham treatment, with minimum of 6 month follow-up, and outcomes of cost, angina frequency/severity/duration, and quality of life improvements. [27] The trial known as MUST-EECP, randomized 139 patients with chronic angina to 35 hours of outpatient therapy with active EECP (n=60) or sham counterpulsation. The results of the trial showed patients in the active EECP therapy group showed a statistically significant increase in time to exercise-induced ST-segment depression and significant decrease in the frequency of angina episodes when compared with sham and baseline over one year. Although this was a positive trial, it must be noted that significantly higher rates (26% vs. 55%) of adverse events, which included leg pain, back pain, and skin abrasions, occurred in the counterpulsation arm.[28] More recent registry data suggest that improvement in symptomatic benefit can be sustained for up to 3 years following treatment. [29]

Transmyocardial Laser Revascularization (TMLR)

TMLR began to be used in 1983 in association with CABG as a complementary technique. [20] Interestingly, the procedure is in part based on reptilian physiology as reptiles do not have significant epicardial coronary circulation. Instead most of their heart's blood supply is delivered directly to heart muscle from the ventricle through a network of channels. The technique is a surgical procedure, usually involving a left thoracotomy. After exposing the heart, a high-energy laser beam is utilized to create channels in the myocardium from the epicardial to the endocardial surface. Initially it was thought that TMLR's mechanism of action was based on direct blood flow to the heart. However, it is now known that these channels close up within two weeks of the procedure. [31] More recent data suggests the possible pathophysiological basis of the procedure involves sympathetic denervation of the myocardium [32] and angiogenesis. [33]

Early on several studies showed TMLR was effective in treating angina, but these were mainly observational studies where the TMLR was not compared to a medicine arm. [34, 35] Subsequently, several RCT's comparing TMLR to medications were published, yet these had mostly contradictory results. The Cochrane Group did a review of these trails and did find that 43.8% of patients in the TMLR group did have significantly improved symptoms, compared with 14.8% in the medication groups. However, the same review found the 30-day mortality as treated was significantly higher at 6.8% in the TMLR group compared 0.8% in the control group. [36] Finally there was one randomized blinded study done with percutaneous TMLR. In this study patients were blinded by being given sedation and dark goggles were placed over the patient's eyes during the entire angioplasty procedure (with or without TMR). This trial showed non-significant improvement of angina class over 6 months. [37] Given the contradictory efficacy results of TMLR study and the significantly higher peri-operative mortality, the use of this technique remains controversial.

Spinal Cord Stimulation (SCS)

SCS was first introduced for the treatment of patients with severe angina pectoris, in the late 1980s. [38] This procedure requires puncturing the epidural space at the level of the fourth or sixth thoracic vertebra, and introducing an electrode to the level of the first or second thoracic vertebra. The electrode is connected to a pulse generator similar to that of a pacemaker which then usually implanted in the anterior abdominal wall. The device can also be programmed like cardiac pacemakers, and/or the patient can use a hand-held programmer to adjust the time and strength of the stimulation received within predetermined boundaries. The mechanism of action for this procedure remains unclear. There is thought that it works via reduced pain perception, decreased sympathetic tone, reduced myocardial oxygen demand, improved coronary microcirculatory blood. [39]

There is a paucity of good large RCT's comparing SCS with a placebo group. A review of the literature done by the Taylor et al, revealed 7 RCT's for a total of 270 patients who have been part of trials comparing SCS to no stimulation and SCS to CABG/TMLR. There was no difference in SCS and CABG/TMLR groups in terms of efficacy. However, in the 5 trials that compared SCS to no stimulation there was a significant improvement in exercise capacity and health-related quality of life of the SCS patient population. In terms of safety concerns of this treatment masking ischemia there were no increases in cardiac morbidity or mortality with SCS when compared to other treatments. Individual trials were small ranging in cohort sizes from 12-15 patients in each arm of the SCS vs. no stimulation trials. [40]

New Pharmacologic Agents

Currently there are many drugs under investigation for use as anti-anginal agents. One class of such drugs includes fatty acid oxidation inhibitors. A medication in this class, trimetazidine, promotes the replacement of fatty acid oxidation to glucose oxidation, thereby increasing cardiac metabolic efficiency. [41] Another novel agent is Nicorandil, a coronary vasodilator with a dual mechanism of action that involves a nitrate-like effect and a potassium ion channel opening action. [42] Finally, ivabradine, a heart rate lowering drug that selectively inhibits the pacemaker current in the sinus node, has also shown promise as an anti-angina agent. [43] All of these medications have been studied in clinical trials but have yet to be approved by the FDA for use in the United States.

Trimetazidine

There have been multiple trials examining the efficacy of Trimetazidine as an anti-angina agent. In one of the largest trials, TRIMPOL II, 426 patients with stable, effort-induced angina and documented CAD who were treated with metoprolol were randomly assigned to trimetazidine or placebo. After 12 weeks, there were significantly greater improvements in the trimetazidine group in time to 1 mm ST segment depression, total workload, time to onset of angina, maximum ST segment depression, mean weekly number of angina attacks, mean weekly nitrate consumption, and grade of anginal pain. [44] Furthermore the Cochrane group did a meta-analysis on 23 trials, for a combined 1378 patients to determine the efficacy and tolerability of trimetazidine in patients with stable angina. The authors concluded a significant reduction in number of weekly angina attacks (mean difference -1.44, $p<0.0001$), reductions in weekly nitroglycerin tablet consumption (mean difference -0.73; $P<0.0001$), and improvement in exercise time to 1 mm segment depression ($P=0.0002$). [45] However, the authors also suggested that a large, long term trial comparing trimetazidine with other anti-anginal drugs assessing clinically relevant important outcomes are required to establish its role in clinical management.

Nicorandil

As a potassium channel activator, nicorandil improves coronary blood flow by dilating the coronary arteries. It is also thought to mimic the natural process of ischemic preconditioning, thus protecting the heart from subsequent ischemic attacks. The largest study investigating nicorandil was the IONA trial, in which 2565 patients were randomized to receive 20 mg of nicorandil twice daily versus 2561patients randomized to receive placebo in addition to standard antianginal therapy. After 1.6 years there was a statistically significant 17% reduction in the combined endpoint of CAD death, nonfatal MI, or unplanned hospital admission for cardiac chest pain in the nicorandil group. [46] The secondary endpoint of CAD and non-fatal myocardial infarction was, however, not significant. Based on this and other studies, nicorandil is approved as an anti-anginal agent in Europe and Japan, but is yet to be approved in the United States.

Ivabradine

Ivabradine is part of a novel class of medications that selectively works on the sinus node to reduce patient heart rates. There have been several studies investigating the efficacy of this medication. In one double-blinded, placebo-controlled trial of 360 patients with chronic stable angina, the ivabradine group had a 12% increase in the time to onset of 1-mm ST-segment depression, and a 9.5% increase in exercise tolerance. [47] The largest trial involving ivabradine was the BEAUTIFUL trial which was a randomized, double-blinded, placebo-controlled study of 10,917 CAD patients with left ventricular ejection fraction < 40%. Patients received ivabradine or placebo in addition to standard medical therapy. There was no significant difference in the primary composite endpoint of cardiovascular death, admission to hospital for acute myocardial infarction, and admission to hospital for new onset or worsening heart failure. However, in the pre-specified subgroup of patients with baseline heart rates of > 70, there was a statistically significant 36% decrease in hospital admissions secondary to fatal and nonfatal MI, and a 30% decrease in coronary revascularization. [48]

Future Directions

One of the more innovative approaches to the treatment of refractory angina is the use of stem cell therapy. One type of such therapy, entails isolating CD34+ cells isolated from bone marrow and then injecting them directly into the coronary arteries percutaneously via catheters. It is thought that these cells may improve perfusion by promoting angiogenesis in both large vessels and the microvasculature thereby reducing symptoms in patients with advanced coronary disease. In one trial in China, 112 patients with refractory angina were randomized to CD34+ versus placebo intracoronary infusion in a double-blinded manner. They found a significant reduction in the frequency of angina episodes per week in the treatment group (−14.6 +/- 4.8 at 3 months and −15.6 +/- 4.0 at 6 months) over the control group (−4.5 +/- 0.3 and −3.0 +/- 1.2, respectively; p < 0.01). [49] Although this therapy is still in its infancy, it has the potential of being a powerful treatment option in the future.

Conclusion

Chronic stable angina is a serious and growing problem among our patient population with a large overall economic impact to society. Traditional strategies of medications and revascularization are the cornerstones of treatment. However, with antiquated trials and guidelines, it is controversial which strategy, revascularization versus medications, is superior first line treatment for both angina relief and mortality benefit. Hopefully, newer studies such as the ISCHEMIA trial will assist in developing a better treatment strategy using current standards of care.

Furthermore, an increasing number of patients with angina presenting to cardiologists are found to be unsuitable for PCI or CABG surgery and continue to experience significant symptoms despite optimal medical therapy. For those patients with "refractory angina", ranolazine should probably be first line treatment and be part of the guidelines. Other strategies such as EECP can also be considered, while there needs to be more studies to prove the efficacy of SCS. The perioperative mortality data of TMLR, however makes it the most risky alternative treatment. Finally newer anti-anginal agents are on the horizon and once FDA approved will likely be a part the treatment plan for angina.

References

[1]   Libby, Peter; Bonnow, Robert; Mann, Douglas; Zipes, Douglas (2007). *Braunwald's Heart Disease: A Textbook of Cardiovascular Medicine.*

[2]   Lloyd-Jones D, Adams RJ, Brown TM, et al. Heart disease and strokestatistics-2010 update: a report from the American Heart Association Statistics Committee and Stroke Statistics Subcommittee. Circulation 2010, 121:e46-e215

[3]   Lloyd-Jones D, Abrams R, Cvarnethon M, et al. Heart disease and stroke statistics-2009 update: a report from the American Heart Association Statistics Committee and Stroke Statistics Subcommittee. *Circulation* 2009;119(3):e21-181.

[4]   Fox K, Garcia MA, Ardissino D, Buszman P, Camici PG, Crea F, et al. Guidelines on the management of stable angina pectoris: executive summary: The Task Force on the Management of Stable Angina Pectoris of the European Society of Cardiology. *Eur Heart J* 2006; 27:1341–1381.

[5]   Patel MR, Dehmer GJ, Hirshfeld JW, Smith PK, Spertus JA. ACCF/SCAI/STS/ AATS/AHA/ASNC 2009 Appropriateness Criteria for Coronary Revascularization: a report by the American College of CardiologyFoundation Appropriateness Criteria Task Force, Society for Cardiovascular Angiography and Interventions, Society of Thoracic Surgeons, American Association for Thoracic Surgery, American Heart Association, and the American Society of Nuclear Cardiology Endorsed by the American Society of Echocardiography, the Heart Failure Society of America, and the Society of Cardiovascular Computed Tomography. *J Am Coll Cardiol* 2009; 53:530–533.

[6]   Diamond GA, Staniloff HM, Forrester JS, et al. Computer-assisted diagnosis in the noninvasive evaluation of patients with suspected coronary disease. *J Am Coll Cardiol* 1983;1:444-55.

[7]   Campeau L. Letter to the editor. *Circulation* 1976;54:522.

[8]   Norton C, Georgiopoulou V, Kalogeropoulos A, and Butler J. Chronic stable angina: pathophysiology and innovations in treatment. *J Cardiovasc Med* (Hagerstown). 2011 Mar;12(3):218-9.

[9]   Gibbons RJ, Abrams J, Chatterjee K, et al. Guidelines for the management of patients with chronic stable angina: a report of the ACC/AHA Task Force on Practice guidelines. *J Am Coll Cardiol* 2007;50(23):2264-74.

[10] Lytle BW, Loop FD, Cosgrove DM, Ratliff NB, Easley K, Taylor PC. Long-term (5 to 12 years) serial studies of internal mammary artery and saphenous vein coronary bypass grafts. *J Thorac Cardiovasc Surg* 1985;89:248-58.

[11] Guidelines and indications for coronary artery bypass graft surgery. A report of the American College of Cardiology/American Heart Association Task Force on Assessment of Diagnostic and Therapeutic Cardiovascular Procedures (Subcommittee on Coronary Artery Bypass Graft Surgery). *J Am Coll Cardiol* 1991;17:543-89.

[12] Holmes DR Jr, Vlietstra RE, Smith HC, et al. Restenosis after percutaneous transluminal coronary angioplasty (PTCA): a report from the PTCA Registry of the National Heart, Lung, and Blood Institute. *Am J Cardiol* 1984;53:77C-81C

[13] Fischman DL, Leon MB, Baim DS, et al. A randomized comparison of coronary-stent placement and balloon angioplasty in the treatment of coronary artery disease. Stent Restenosis Study Investigators. *N Engl J Med* 1994;331:496-501.

[14] Maarten L. Simoons and Stephan Windecker Chronic stable coronary artery disease: drugs vs. revascularization, *European Heart Journal* (2010) 31, 530–541

[15] Frye RL, August P, Brooks MM, Hardison RM, Kelsey SF, MacGregor JM, Orchard TJ, Chaitman BR, Genuth SM, Goldberg SH, Hlatky MA, Jones TL, Molitch ME, Nesto RW, Sako EY, Sobel BE. A randomized trial of therapies for type 2 diabetes and coronary artery disease. *N Engl J Med* 2009;360: 2503–2515.

[16] Boden WE, O'Rourke RA, Teo KK, et al. Optimal medical therapy with or without PCI for stable coronary disease. *N Engl J Med* 2007;356:1503-16.

[17] New York University. NIH awards $84 million grant to NYU Langone Medical Center and partnering institutions for first-of-its-kind comparative effectiveness ischemia clinical trial [press release]. August 1, 2011.

[18] St Jude Medical. Independent data safety monitoring board recommends St Jude Medical's FAME II clinical trial stop enrollment following positive interim analysis *[press release]*. January 18, 2012

[19] Mannheimer C, Camici P, Chester MR, et al. The problem of chronic refractory angina; report from the ESC Joint Study Group on the Treatment of Refractory *Angina. Eur Heart J* 2002; 23:355–370.

[20] Gibbons RJ, Abrams J, Chatterjee K, et al. Guidelines for the management of patients with chronic stable angina: a report of the ACC/AHA Task Force on Practice guidelines. *J Am Coll Cardiol* 2007;50(23):2264-74.

[21] MacInnes A, Fairman DA, Binding P, Rhodes JA, Wyatt MJ, Phelan A, Haddock PS, Karran EH. The antianginal agent trimetazidine does not exert its functional benefit via inhibition of mitochondrial long-chain 3-ketoacyl coenzyme A thiolase. *Circ Res.* 2003;93:e26–e32.

[22] Belardinelli L, Antzelevitch C, Fraser H. Inhibition of late (sustained/persistent) sodium current: a potential drug target to reduce intracellular sodium-dependent calcium overload and its detrimental effects on cardiomyocyte function. *Eur Heart J.* 2004;6(suppl I):I3–I7.

[23] Palaniswamy C and Aronow W. Treatment of Stable Angina Pectoris. *American Journal of Therapeutics* 18, e138–e152 (2011).

[24] Chaitman BR, Pepine CJ, Parker JO, et al. Effects of ranolazine with atenolol, amlodipine, or diltiazem on exercise tolerance and angina frequency in patients with severe chronic angina: a randomized controlled trial. *JAMA* 2004;291:309-16.

[25] Morrow DA, Scirica BM, Karwatowska-Prokopczuk E et al.;MERLIN-TIMI 36 Trial Investigators. Effects of ranolazine on recurrent cardiovascular events in patients with non-ST-elevation acute coronary syndromes: The MERLIN-TIMI 36 randomized trial. *JAMA,* 2007; 297: 1775–1783.

[26] Kantrowitz A, Kantrowitz A. Experimental augmentation of coronary flow by retardation of coronary artery pressure pulse. *Surgery* 1953;34:678–87.

[27] Amin F, AlHajeri A, Civelek B, Fedorowicz Z,Manzer BM. Enhanced external counterpulsation for chronic angina pectoris. *Cochrane Database of Systematic Reviews 2010,* Issue 2. Art. No.: CD007219. DOI: 10.1002/14651858.CD007219.pub2.

[28] Arora RR, Chou TM, Jain D, et al. The Multicenter Study of Enhanced External Counterpulsation (MUST-EECP): effect of EECP on exercise-induced myocardial ischemia and anginal episodes. *J Am Coll Cardiol* 1999;33:1833– 40.

[29] Loh PH, Cleland JG, Louis AA, et al. Enhanced external counterpulsation in the treatment of chronic refractory angina: a long-term follow-up outcome from the International Enhanced External Counterpulsation Patient Registry. *Clin Cardiol* 2008; 31:159–164.

[30] Smith JA, Dunning JJ, Parry AJ, Large SR, Wallwork J. Transmyocardial laser revascularization. *Journal of Cardiac Surgery* 1995;10(5):569–72.

[31] Fisher PE, Khomoto T, DeRosa CM, et al. Histologic analysis of transmyocardial channels: comparison of $CO2$ and Holmium:YAG lasers. *Ann Thorac Surg.* 1997;64:466–472.

[32] Al-Sheikh T, Allen KB, Straka SP, et al. Cardiac sympathetic denervation after transmyocardial laser revascularization. *Circulation.* 1999; 100:135–140.

[33] Horvath KA, Chiu E, Maun DC, et al. Up-regulation of vascular endothelial growth factor mRNA and angiogenesis after transmyocardial laser revascularization. *Ann Thorac Surg.* 1999;68:825–829.

[34] Cooley DA, Frazier OH, Kadipasaoglu KA, Lindenmeir MH, Pehlivanoglu S, Kolff JW, et al.Transmyocardial laser revascularization: clinical experience with twelve-month follow-up. *Journal of Thoracic and Cardiovascular Surgery* 1996;111:791–7.

[35] Frazier OH, Cooley DA, Kadipasaoglu KA, Pehlivanoglu S, Lindenmeir MH, Barasch E, et al.Myocardial revascularization with laser: preliminary findings. *Circulation* 1995;92(Suppl II):58–65.

[36] Briones E, Lacalle JR,Marin I. Transmyocardial laser revascularization versusmedical therapy for refractory angina. *Cochrane Database of Systematic Reviews* 2009, Issue 1. Art. No.: CD003712. DOI: 10.1002/14651858.CD003712.pub2.

[37] Stone GW, Teirstein PS, Rubenstein R, et al. A prospective, multicenter, randomized trial of percutaneous transmyocardial laser revascularization in patients with nonrecanalizable chronic total occlusions. *J Am Coll Cardiol.* 2002;39:1581–1587.

[38] Murphy DF, Giles KE. Dorsal column stimulation for pain relief from intractable angina pectoris. *Pain* 1987;28:365–8.

[39] Latif OA, Nedeljkovic SS, Stevenson LW. Spinal cord stimulation for chronic intractable angina pectoris: a unified theory on its mechanism. *Clin Cardiol* 2001; 24: 533-41.

[40] Taylor RS, De Vries J, Buchser E and DeJongste M. Spinal cord stimulation in the treatment of refractory angina: systematic review and meta-analysis of randomized controlled trials *BMC Cardiovascular Disorders* 2009, **9**:13.

[41] Morrow DA, Givertz MM. Modulation of myocardial energetics: emerging evidence for a therapeutic target in cardiovascular disease. *Circulation* 2005; 112:3280-3288.

[42] Taira N. Nicorandil as a hybrid between nitrates and potassium channel activators. *J Cardiol.* 1989;63:J18–J24.

[43] DiFrancesco CD, Camm JA. Heart rate lowering by specific and selective If current inhibition with ivabradine. A new therapeutic perspective in cardiovascular disease. *Drugs.* 2004;64:1757–1765.

[44] Szwed H, Sadowski Z, Elikowski W, et al. Combination treatment in stable effort angina using trimetazidine and metoprolol: results of a randomized, double-blind, multicentre study (TRIMPOL II). TRIMetazidine in POLand. *Eur Heart J* 2001; 22: 2267-2274.

[45] Ciapponi A, Pizarro R, Harrison J. Trimetazidine for stable angina. *Cochrane Database Syst Rev* 2005; :CD003614.

[46] The IONA Study Group. Effect of nicorandil on coronary events in patients with stable angina: the Impact of Nicorandil in Angina (IONA) randomized trial. *Lancet.* 2002;359:1269–1275.

[47] Borer JS, Fox K, Jaillon P, Lerebours G; Ivabradine Investigators Group. Antianginal and anti-ischemic effects of ivabradine, an I(f) inhibitor, in stable angina: A randomized, double-blind, multicentre, placebo-controlled trial. *Circulation,* 2003; 107: 817–823.

[48] Fox K, Ford I, Steg PG, et al. Ivabradine for patients with stable coronary artery disease and left-ventricular systolic dysfunction (BEAUTIFUL): a randomized, double-blind, placebo-controlled trial. *Lancet* 2008; 372:807-816.

[49] Wang S, Cui J, Peng W, and Lu M. Intracoronary Autologous CD34+ Stem Cell Therapy for Intractable Angina. *Cardiology* 2010;117:140–147.

In: Current Issues in the Management of Stable Ischemic Heart …   ISBN: 978-1-62417-203-8
Editor: Mukesh Singh   © 2013 Nova Science Publishers, Inc.

Chapter VI

Current Understanding in Pathophysiology and Management of Cardiac Syndrome X

Hardeep Kaur Grewal, Manish Bansal and Ravi R. Kasliwal[*]
Medanta - The Medicity, Gurgaon, Haryana, India

Abstract

Harvey Kemp in 1973 coined the term 'syndrome X' to refer to a syndrome of typical exertional angina pectoris, positive exercise ECG stress test and angiographically normal epicardial coronary arteries where other cardiac and systemic diseases known to affect vascular function had been ruled out. Later, this term was changed to 'cardiac syndrome X' (CSX). Although, over the past three decades, considerable advancements have been made in the understanding of the pathophysiology of CSX, it still remains a major diagnostic and therapeutic challenge. Not only is it difficult to establish the correct diagnosis, the treatment of this condition is also less rewarding. Consequently, CSX continues to be a source of significant morbidity and mental agony for the patients and substantial healthcare expenditure for the system. The present review discusses the current understanding of the pathophysiology of CSX and presents a practical approach for evaluation and management of the patients presenting with this condition.

Introduction

It was long believed that angina pectoris occurred almost invariably as a consequence of obstructive disease, or less commonly, spasm of the large coronary arteries. However, with

---

[*] Corresponding author. Ravi R Kasliwal, Chairman, Clinical and Preventive Cardiology, # 9, 3rd Floor OPD, Medanta- The Medicity, Sector 38, Gurgaon, Haryana- 122001, India. Ph: +91-124-4141414; Fax: +91-124-4834111; Email: rrkasliwal@hotmail.com.

the advent of coronary angiography, it was soon realized that a substantial proportions of patients presented with typical angina chest pain did not have any significant coronary atherosclerosis [1,2]. Indeed, almost 20-30% of the patients undergoing coronary angiography for suspected coronary artery disease (CAD) actually turn out to have apparently 'normal' coronary arteries [1,3]. Harvey Kemp in 1973 coined the term 'syndrome X' to encompass this group of patients [4]. The term was used to refer to a syndrome of typical exertional angina pectoris, positive exercise ECG stress test and angiographically normal epicardial coronary arteries where other cardiac and systemic diseases known to affect vascular function had been ruled out. Later this term was changed to 'cardiac syndrome X' (CSX) to differentiate it from a more common metabolic syndrome X, which was a constellation of multiple metabolic abnormalities, commonly seen in obese individuals.

Although, over the past three decades, considerable advancements have been made in the understanding of the pathophysiology of CSX, it still remains a major diagnostic and therapeutic challenge. Not only it is difficult to establish the correct diagnosis, the treatment of this condition is also less rewarding. Consequently, CSX continues to be a source of significant morbidity and mental agony for the patients and substantial healthcare expenditure for the system. The present review discusses the current understanding of the pathophysiology of CSX and presents a practical approach for evaluation and management of the patients presenting with this condition.

Pathogenesis of CSX

Despite extensive research, pathogenesis of CSX remains a matter of considerable debate. However, the expert opinion seems to converge mainly on two mechanisms- microvascular dysfunction (MVD) resulting in myocardial perfusion abnormalities or ischemia and heightened cardiac pain perception [5-7].

Evidence of Myocardial Ischemia

Right from the initial description of CSX by Kemp, development of typical ischemic ECG changes during exercise stress test has been the fundamental criterion for diagnosis of CSX. In addition to exercise, these ECG abnormalities have been reported in response to other forms of cardiac stressors also, such as rapid atrial pacing and intravenous infusion of dobutamine, dipyridamole and adenosine [8,9]. Furthermore, as documented on Holter monitoring, ST-segment changes in patients with CSX are known to occur during spontaneous episodes of chest pain also [10-12].

Though development of ECG changes during stress may suggest myocardial ischemia as the underlying mechanism, such changes may also be false-positive. Accordingly, more definitive and direct evidence of ischemia has been sought in various studies. In a retrospective review of data, Tweddel et al demonstrated perfusion defects on stress thallium scintigraphy in 98 of 100 patients with angina and normal coronary arteriograms [13]. Similarly, Lanza et al found dobutamine induced gadolinium defects suggestive of subendocardial ischemia on cardiac magnetic resonance imaging (MRI) in a significant proportion of patients with CSX [5]. Other investigators have tried to look for metabolic abnormalities to document occurrence of myocardial ischemia in these patients. Increased myocardial lactate and isoprostane production, coronary sinus oxygen desaturation and coronary sinus pH reduction have been demonstrated in $\geq$20% patients with CSX [14]. Buffon et al measured levels of lipid hydroperoxides and conjugated dienes as metabolic markers of ischemia in great cardiac vein [15]. Following rapid atrial pacing, there was significant increase in the levels of these markers in patients with CSX but not in control subjects. In majority of these patients, the metabolic alterations occurred concurrently with the development of ischemic ST-segment changes and chest pain. In the WISE (women's Ischemia Syndrome Evaluation) study, 7 of the 35 women with features of CSX who underwent phospohorus-31 nuclear magnetic resonance (NMR) spectroscopy had typical metabolic findings of myocardial ischemia during repetitive handgrip exercise [16].

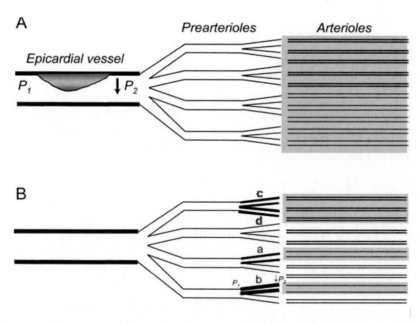

Figure 1. Differences in myocardial ischemia resulting from a significant stenosis in an epicardial coronary artery (A) or from coronary microvascular dysfunction (B). In the case of an epicardial stenosis, entire myocardial territory supplied by that artery gets affected resulting in a large area of ischemia (shaded area). In contrast, in the case of microvascular dysfunction, small areas of myocardial ischemia occur which are patchily distributed throughout the myocardium. a, b c and d indicate dysfunctional microvessels; P1 and P2, blood pressure proximal and distal to the diseased vessels. Modified from reference [19].

Thus, it is apparent that myocardial ischemia does indeed play an important role in the pathogenesis of CSX. However, the evidence of myocardial ischemia in patients with CSX has not always been so forthcoming. Most notable has been the consistent lack of inducible wall motion abnormalities on stress echocardiography in these patients [17,18]. The patients with CSX fail to develop wall motion abnormalities in response to exercise or pharmacological stress despite development of significant ECG changes and chest pain. This finding has been used as an argument to suggest that myocardial ischemia is not the predominant mechanism responsible for symptoms in these patients. This is further supported by the fact that even the metabolic evidence of myocardial ischemia, as described above, can be demonstrated in only 20-25% patients with CSX [14, 16). However, it must be noted that, unlike the patients with obstructive CAD, coronary blood flow (CBF) abnormalities in patients with CSX do not uniformly involve all coronary microvessels of a major coronary branch. Rather, the coronary involvement in CSX is typically patchy and is scattered all over the myocardium (figure 1) [19]. Consequently, the resulting perfusion abnormalities are not large enough to produce wall motion abnormalities on echocardiography, even though they may be sufficient enough to cause chest pain and ECG changes. The same phenomenon can also explain why the metabolic evidence of myocardial ischemia is not detectable in all the patients with CSX. The metabolites released from the ischemic myocardium get diluted by the blood coming from the normal, non-ischemic myocardium and therefore the levels of these metabolites in the coronary sinus or its main tributaries fail to meet the diagnostic criteria for myocardial ischemia.

Evidence of Microvascular Dysfunction

As the patients with CSX do not have obstructive CAD on coronary angiograms, abnormalities of coronary microcirculation have been proposed as the mechanism underlying development of myocardial ischemia, ECG changes and chest pain in these patients. Studies using various invasive and non-invasive modalities have demonstrated impaired CBF response to various coronary vasodilator stimuli in these patients [20]. Bottcher et al studied 25 women with CSX using myocardial positron emission tomography (PET) and reported a blunted increase in CBF in response to dipyridamole [20-25]. A similar blunted CBF response to dipyridamole had earlier been shown by Opherk et al also, using argon washout method for measuring CBF [22]. In the WISE study, 74 of the 159 women undergoing invasive study had subnormal coronary flow response to intracoronary adenosine [23]. Likewise, a number of studies have shown impaired coronary flow reserve (CFR) in response to intracoronary injection of acetylcholine- a potent coronary vasodilator [24,25]. Motz et al measured coronary flow in response to acetylcholine and dipyridamole in 23 patients with clinically suspected CAD and normal coronary arteries on angiogram [24]. CBF was measured using the argon washout method. Acetylcholine failed to increase CBF in 14 of these 23 patients and resulted in paradoxical vasoconstriction in another 3 of them. In yet another study, Egashira et al reported that intracoronary injection of increasing doses of acetylcholine caused a lower dose-dependent increase in CBF in patients with CSX as compared to the controls [25].

In addition to the impaired response to coronary vasodilator stimuli, the patients with CSX also exhibit exaggerated response to coronary vasoconstrictor agents such as intravenous ergonovine [26]. Moreover, as mentioned above, intracoronary acetylcholine has been shown to induce paradoxical vasoconstriction with consequent CBF reduction in many patients with CSX [24].

Mechanisms of Microvascular Dysfunction

A number of mechanisms have been proposed to explain coronary microcirculatory abnormalities seen in patients with CSX. These include endothelial dysfunction, altered autonomic tone, insulin resistance, inflammation, estrogen deficiency, abnormalities of ion-flux, altered rheological properties, etc.

Role of Endothelium

Endothelium is regarded as the gatekeeper of vascular health [27]. The endothelial cells produce several mediators such as nitric oxide, prostacyclin, C-type natriuretic peptide, etc. that have vasorelaxant, anti-proliferative, antithrombotic, and anti-adherent effects [27-29]. Among these, nitric oxide appears to be most important molecule, mediating most of the vasculoprotective effects of the endothelium. However, at the same time, endothelial cells also produce substances with opposing effects such as endothelin, thromboxane A2, prostaglandin H2, and oxygen free radicals. The release of these substances is controlled in such a manner that in health, vasculoprotective effects predominate. However, with impairment of endothelial function, there is reduced production and release of vasculoprotective substances, particularly nitric oxide, resulting in increased susceptibility to vascular injury leading to progressive vascular damage [27,30].

Several studies have provided strong evidence to support the role of endothelial dysfunction in causation of coronary microcirculatory abnormalities seen in patients with CSX [25,31-34]. The patients with CSX are reported to have lower circulatory levels of nitric oxide and higher levels of endothelin-1 [32,33]. Transient myocardial perfusion defects have been reported in areas supplied by arteries showing endothelial dysfunction [31]. Intracoronary acetylcholine, an endothelium-dependent coronary vasodilator, often produces paradoxical vasoconstriction with consequent reduction in CBF in patients with CSX, as described above. Furthermore, the vasodilatory response to acetylcholine is normalized by the administration of L-arginine (the substrate for nitric oxide synthesis) and tetrahydrobiopterin (a nitric oxide synthase cofactor), lending further support to the role of endothelial dysfunction in the development of these abnormalities [34]. Finally, as demonstrated by studies using brachial artery flow-mediated dilatation, the patients with CSX are also more likely to have evidence of endothelial dysfunction in the peripheral vascular beds [35,36].

The endothelial dysfunction in CSX appears to be multi-factorial in origin [30]. Hypertension, diabetes, smoking, obesity and hypercholesterolemia are known potent mediators of endothelial dysfunction. Although, the earlier definition of CSX had excluded hypertensives and diabetics, the syndrome of angina with normal coronary arteries occurs commonly in patients with hypertension and diabetes. Accordingly, several investigators have advocated that these patients should also be included in the definition of CSX [5]. In addition, insulin resistance itself, in absence of diabetes can lead to endothelial dysfunction and may contribute to the MVD observed in patients with CSX [37,38]. A blunted nitric oxide and endothelin responsiveness to intravenously infused insulin has been reported in patients with angina pectoris and angiographically normal coronary arteries [38]. Moreover, interventions known to improve insulin sensitivity have been shown to improve microvascular endothelial function and decrease myocardial ischemia in patients with CSX [39].

Given the high prevalence (approximately 70% in most series) of postmenopausal women in the CSX population, estrogen deficiency has also been postulated as a pathogenic agent causing MVD. Estrogen deficiency can act via both the endothelium-dependent and the endothelium-independent mechanisms [40]. Indeed, the administration of 17β-estradiol has been shown to improve coronary endothelial function and decrease exercise induced angina and frequency of chest pain in postmenopausal women with CSX [41-43]. Finally, inflammation, as described below, can act both as a marker as well as the mediator of endothelial dysfunction in patients with CSX.

Role of Inflammation

Numerous studies in patients with atherosclerotic vascular disease have firmly established the role of inflammation in the initiation and progression of atherosclerosis [44]. Similar pathogenic mechanism may operate in patients with CSX also, resulting in MVD. Several authors have reported increased concentrations of circulating C-reactive protein (CRP) – an acute-phase reactant and a marker of chronic inflammation and vascular disease – that correlate well with vascular abnormalities in patients with CSX [10,45,46]. In a study on 137 consecutive patients with typical chest pain and normal coronary angiograms, Cosin-Sales et al found higher CRP concentrations among those with frequent and prolonged episodes of chest pain or those with ST-segment depression on exercise test or Holter monitoring [10]. In contrast, the patients with shorter episodes of chest pain, negative exercise stress test and no ST-segment shifts on Holter monitoring had much lower concentrations of CRP. Moreover, CRP was found to be the only independent predictor of abnormal findings on Holter monitoring and exercise testing in this study. In yet another study, CRP levels were found to predict CBF response to intracoronary acetylcholine injection [45].

Other Pathogenic Mechanisms

Nearly three-fourth of all patients with CSX are known to have impaired cardiac uptake of metaiodobenzylguanidine (MIBG), indicating abnormal handling of norepinephrine in the cardiac sympathetic nerve endings [47]. Although the exact significance of this finding is not known, it is suggested that this may contribute to MVD seen in these patients.

The patients with CSX are also known to have rheological abnormalities such as increased red blood cell aggregation, elevated hematocrit-corrected blood viscosity, plasma viscosity, etc. These factors may induce myocardial perfusion disturbances by adversely affecting blood flow in the coronary microcirculation [48].

Lastly, increased membrane Na^+/H^+ exchanger activity, the major regulator of intracellular pH and consequently the cellular Ca^{2+} handling, has also been described in patients with CSX. Abnormally increased intracellular calcium concentrations can favour vasoconstriction and may compromise myocardial blood circulation [49].

Abnormal Cardiac Pain Perception

Several clinical observations have suggested that abnormal pain perception may be the fundamental abnormality in a sizeable proportion of the patients with CSX. Characteristic chest pain can be induced by manoeuvres, which are otherwise painless, such as injection of saline in to right atrium, intra-cardiac catheter manipulation or contrast injection in to the left coronary artery (figure 2) [8,50,51]. Similarly, in patients with CSX, ventricular pacing at a slow rate (only 5 beats faster than the resting heart rate) has been shown to provoke typical chest pain with the pain worsening with the increasing stimulus intensity [8,51]. Lastly, cardiac stress testing with dobutamine, adenosine and dipyridamole often causes severe chest pain in these patients despite the absence of inducible wall motion abnormalities whereas the pain is much less marked in patients with obstructive CAD who have readily detectable myocardial ischemia on echocardiography [9].

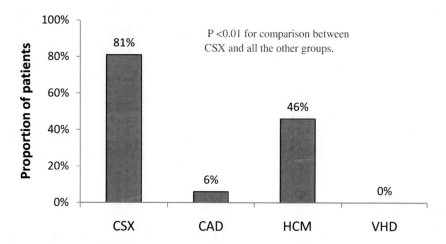

Figure 2. Proportion of patients, with different cardiac conditions, experiencing chest pain during cardiac catheterization. The chest pain was provoked by right ventricular pacing at 5 beats over resting heart rate and/or by injection of contrast medium into the left coronary artery. CAD- coronary artery disease; CSX-cardiac syndrome X, HCM- hypertrophic cardiomyopathy, VHD- valvular heart disease. Modified from reference [8].

The exaggerated pain sensitivity in patients with CSX has been documented in response to several non-cardiac stimuli also, such as esophageal stimulation, electrical skin stimulation, forearm ischemia, etc [52,53]. However, it is important to note that these observations have been made mostly from the non-randomized studies. The data from more controlled studies suggests that the heightened pain perception in patients with CSX is related primarily to cardiac stimuli only [8].

The mechanisms responsible for this exaggerated pain sensitivity have not been fully elucidated. Rosen et al used PET scan to measure regional cerebral blood flow during dobutamine stress testing in 8 patients with CSX and 8 controls [54]. They found a significant increase in blood flow in right insula in CSX patients but not in controls. The same group, in a previous study, had already demonstrated a lack of right insular activation during dobutamine stress in patients with obstructive CAD [55]. Together, these findings imply that the central modulation of pain is probably abnormal in patients with CSX. Based on such observations, it has been proposed that the CSX patients likely have an ineffective thalamic gate that allows inappropriate cortical activation by afferent stimuli from the heart, resulting in increased pain perception. Accordingly, spinal cord stimulation, which is believed to augment pain-gate control in the dorsal horn, has been reported to improve anginal symptoms in patients with CSX [56]. Other studies have, however, suggested that the abnormality resides primarily within the cardiac afferent fibres themselves. This argument is supported by the finding of improper cardiac adrenergic nerve function, as detected by cardiac MIBG scintigraphy, in patients with CSX [47,57]. Excessive release of potassium, adenosine and endothelin-1 and the abnormal responses by the endogenous opioid system have also been postulated to play role in augmented pain perception in some patients [58].

Abnormal cardiac pain perception in presence of coronary microvascular dysfunction: The final common pathway

Irrespective of the relative significance of different mechanisms in induction of chest pain in patients with CSX, it appears that in vast majority of these patients, both MVD and the enhanced pain perception operate together. The combined effects of MVD, leading to minor reductions in myocardial blood flow, and increased pain perception may explain the prolonged, severe episodes of typical chest pain which are usually out of proportion to the extent of ischemia.

Multiple theories have been proposed to link MVD with exaggerated pain sensitivity in patients with CSX. It is suggested that repeated subclinical episodes of myocardial ischemia may themselves damage cardiac nerve fibres resulting in increased response to otherwise painless stimuli [57]. Alternately, a primary abnormality of cardiac nerve fibres itself can lead to both the increased pain perception (afferent fibres) and the MVD (efferent fibres). Lastly, a common pathological process (such as inflammation) may separately but simultaneously affect coronary microvascular and cardiac nerve function.

Diagnostic Approach

Establishing the diagnosis of CSX in clinical practice is a challenging task. This relates both to a lack of consensus on the exact underlying pathogenic mechanism of CSX as well as to the complexities involved in documenting coronary MVD. Therefore, in practice, the diagnosis of CSX is established primarily by exclusion, in the presence of appropriate clinical setting (11.3). However, a systematic, step-by-step approach is helpful in avoiding unwarranted investigations and in reaching the accurate diagnosis.

What is required to establish a diagnosis of CSX?

The initial definition of CSX required presence of angina chest pain, ischemic ECG changes during the stress test, normal epicardial coronary arteries on angiogram and absence of any condition which could affect coronary arterial structure and function. However, this definition had certain limitations. All patients with CSX may not necessarily develop typical ECG changes on stress testing despite having evidence of coronary MVD. Secondly, several atherosclerotic risk factors such as hypertension, diabetes, smoking, dyslipidemia can produce typical clinical presentation of CSX, without resulting in development of stenotic lesions in the coronary arteries. Since the underlying pathophysiology and the treatment approach for these patients is same as that for those with the classical form of CSX, excluding such patients from the definition of CSX does not serve any diagnostic or therapeutic purpose. To address these issues, Lanza and the group have proposed a modified definition of CSX, which appears to be more relevant to the day-to-day clinical practice [5]. According to this definition, a diagnosis of CSX requires the following-

- Typical stable angina, exclusively or predominantly induced by effort
- Findings compatible with myocardial ischemia or coronary MVD on diagnostic investigation including one or more of the following:
    1) diagnostic ST-segment depression during spontaneous or stress-induced typical chest pain;

2) reversible perfusion defects on stress myocardial scintigraphy;

3) documentation of stress-related CBF abnormalities by more advanced diagnostic techniques [e.g. Cardiac MRI, PET scan, Doppler ultrasound, etc.]; and

4) metabolic evidence of transient myocardial ischemia (cardiac PET or MRI or invasive assessment).

- Normal (or near normal) coronary arteries on angiography, and

- Absence of any other specific cardiac disease (eg, variant angina, cardiomyopathy, valvular disease, etc.) but cardiovascular (CV) risk factors such as hypertension, diabetes, etc. are not excluded.

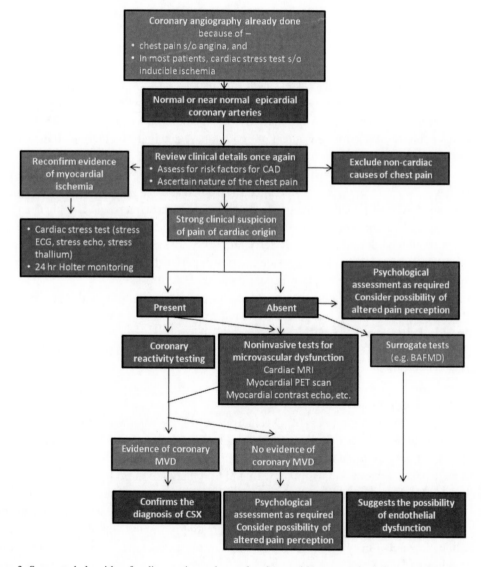

Figure 3. Suggested algorithm for diagnostic work-up of patients with suspected cardiac syndrome X. BAFMD- brachial artery flow-mediated vasodilatation; CAD- coronary artery disease; CSX- cardiac syndrome X; ECG- electrocardiography; MRI- magnetic resonance imaging; MVD- microvascular dysfunction; PET- positron emission tomography; and s/o- suggestive of.

In most patients, the question of CSX arises only after the coronary angiogram (conventional or computed tomographic) has already been done for the evaluation of typical anginal chest pain and, unexpectedly, no significant stenotic lesion has been found in the epicardial coronary arteries. It is then that the search for an alternative mechanism to explain the symptoms begins and CSX becomes a possibility. At this stage, one has to first thoroughly review the clinical details and the stress test findings to ensure that the symptoms were indeed 'real'. Non-cardiac causes of chest pain need to be looked for and carefully excluded. Subsequently, in most patients, some form of diagnostic testing will be required to assess the coronary microvascular function and to document MVD, if present. At the same time, in many patients, psychological assessment will also be called for to uncover a behaviour pattern that would suggest high likelihood of CSX (figure 3).

Clinical Assessment

The major goals of the clinical assessment in a patient suspected to be having CSX are- 1) to ascertain whether the clinical presentation is commensurate with the diagnosis of CSX, 2) to evaluate the presence of conventional CV risk factors and 3) to rule out other disease states which could result in similar clinical presentation. A detailed psychological/ psychiatric assessment, as described below, is also warranted in many patients.

CSX is more common in women than in men. The vast majority of the patients (approximately 70%) are peri- or post-menopausal women and are younger than usual age for atherosclerotic CAD [40]. Although, in most patients the chest pain has a typical anginal character, atypical features are also not uncommon. Thus, the chest pain may develop at rest, may have a prolonged duration and may respond poorly to the administration of sublingual nitrate [59]. During stress test also, the patients may experience severe chest pain which can persist for prolonged periods even after discontinuation of the stress.

An important objective of clinical assessment in patients presenting with chest pain but having normal coronary arteries is to look for and exclude the non-cardiac causes of chest pain. Musculoskeletal disorders, respiratory diseases, gastrointestinal disorders can all cause chest pain and can be identified by a careful clinical examination, supplemented by appropriate diagnostic investigations.

Psychological Aspects

CSX patients have high rates of psychiatric morbidity- approximately 30% have a treatable psychiatric disorder and another 30% have psychological problems. It is observed that the CSX patients are often anxious, have higher incidence of panic disorder and are more likely to be depressed than normals [60,61]. In addition, they are more likely than controls to feel exhausted, to hyperventilate and to somatise their symptoms [62]. These patients have greater level of worry about their illness and many times fail to be reassured even by the finding of a normal coronary arteriogram. Interestingly, many of these behavioural abnormalities have also been shown to correlate with the extent of ST segment changes on Holter monitoring [12].

Thorough psychological assessment in patients with suspected CSX may aid in diagnosis by identifying patient subsets that are likely substrate for CSX. In addition, psychological assessment may also be helpful during the treatment of these patients as suboptimal response is common, leading to significant amount of anxiety, frustration and depression.

Stress Tests

As discussed above, in most patients with suspected CSX, stress test is already done by the time CSX is considered a diagnostic possibility. In such patients, when the obstructive CAD has been ruled out on coronary angiogram, a careful review of the initial stress test findings is required as the first step. In many of them, a repeat stress testing (same or a different modality) may also be called for to gain additional insights in to the pathophysiological mechanisms responsible for the patients' symptoms. It is therefore important to know the characteristics and the relative merits of different stress test methodologies in patients with CSX.

Exercise stress ECG is usually the first-choice stress test performed in most patients presenting with chest pain. The development of significant ST segment depression or elevation during exercise is considered to be a marker of inducible ischemia and usually indicates presence of obstructive CAD. Significant ECG changes are known to occur in patients with CSX as well and may be almost indistinguishable from those seen in patients with obstructive CAD. However, there are certain features that can point towards the possibility of CSX. In patients with CSX, ST-segment depression is usually seen at a higher rate pressure product [63]. These ECG changes are often accompanied by severe chest pain which persists for several minutes after the exercise is stopped and shows poor or slow response to sublingual nitroglycerine [59]. In addition, pre-medication with sublingual nitrate can also help in distinguishing between angina due to MVA and due to obstructive CAD. Repeating exercise testing after giving sublingual nitrates usually improves exercise-induced ECG changes and symptoms in patients with CAD, whereas in patients with CSX, the ECG changes may paradoxically worsen and appear earlier during the test [64].

Although the development of significant ECG changes during exercise has always been considered to be a pre-requisite for diagnosing CSX, it has been learnt over the years that a sizeable proportion of patients with CSX do not actually develop these typical ECG changes [5]. An alternate evidence of myocardial ischemia may be warranted in such patients. Stress nuclear scintigraphy is a commonly employed modality for this purpose, though the accuracy of stress nuclear scintigraphy for detection of myocardial ischemia in patients with CSX remains debatable [65-69]. Overall, approximately 30% patients with CSX show transient perfusion abnormalities compatible with myocardial ischemia on thallium-201 scintigraphy [65,66,69]. Unlike the obstructive CAD, a diffuse, patchy involvement is common in these patients and indicates the possibility of underlying MVD. In addition, majority of the patients with CSX show significantly lower thallium-201 uptake and slower washout kinetics, even if the scan is grossly normal [70].

Stress echocardiography is another commonly utilized technique for detection of myocardial ischemia in patients presenting with chest pain. However, for the reasons discussed above, stress echocardiography consistently fails to show inducible wall motion abnormality in patients with CSX [17,18]. Indeed, occurrence of angina and ST-segment depression in the absence of inducible wall motion abnormalities during dipyridamole or dobutamine stress echocardiography is highly suggestive of microvascular origin of symptoms and is considered to be the hallmark of CSX.

Ambulatory ECG Monitoring

In many patients with CSX, significant ST-segment changes can be recorded during the spontaneous episodes of chest pain on 24-hour Holter monitoring [10-12]. In addition, the extent of ST-segment changes on 24-hour Holter monitoring has been shown to correlate with the severity of chest discomfort, anxiety scores and the circulating levels of CRP in these patients [10].

Thus, 24-hour Holter monitoring can be a useful investigation in patients with CSX, particularly when the clinical suspicion is high and the stress testing has been normal. It can document evidence of ongoing myocardial ischemia and also provide symptoms-ECG correlation.

Coronary Angiography

As is implicit in the definition of CSX, a coronary angiogram documenting absence of obstructive CAD is must before a diagnosis of CSX can be entertained. However, hemodynamically insignificant plaques may be present in many of these patients.

Invasive Evaluation of Coronary Blood Flow (Table 1)

As the patients with CSX present with clinical features highly suggestive of ischemic heart disease but the coronary angiogram is normal, an alternate mechanism to explain the symptoms need to be searched for and demonstrated. Since MVD is one of the key underlying abnormalities, an assessment of coronary microvascular function is often required to establish the diagnosis of CSX with certainty. Traditionally, the assessment of coronary microvascular function is done in the cardiac catheterization laboratory [71]. Intra-coronary Doppler measurement of CBF following intracoronary injection of acetylcholine is the current gold-standard for this purpose. If acetylcholine is not available, other coronary vasodilators such as intracoronary papavarine or intravenous infusion of dipyridamole or adenosine can also be employed. Similarly, thermodilution or argon washout methods can be used for measuring CBF response when intracoronary Doppler wire is not available.

Although the invasive assessment is the most accurate method for demonstrating coronary MVD, there are inherent complexities (need of expertise, cost considerations, risk of complications such as coronary dissection, etc.) involved in these methods limiting their routine use. The best opportunity to perform these tests is at the time of initial coronary angiogram. It may be a good idea to routinely proceed with one of the above methods to document coronary MVD when no significant CAD is found on coronary angiogram in a patient who has presented with typical chest pain and has abnormal stress test.

Table 1. Commonly used modalities for assessment of microvascular function in coronary and peripheral circulation

Stressor/ stimulus	Assessment modality	Remarks
Coronary circulation		
Intracoronary acetylcholine or papavarine	Intracoronary Doppler	The current 'gold-standard' for this purpose but is invasive
Intravenous dipyridamole/ adenosine	Thermodilution Argon wash-out	Invasive, technical difficulties
Intravenous dipyridamole/ adenosine	• Magnetic resonance imaging • Positron emission tomography	Non-invasive; Cardiac magnetic resonance imaging is emerging as a promising modality for this purpose
Intravenous dipyridamole/ adenosine	Doppler echocardiographic estimation of coronary blood flow	Limited feasibility, applicable only to left anterior descending artery territory
Intravenous dipyridamole/ adenosine	Myocardial contrast echocardiography	Non-invasive, allows simultaneous assessment of cardiac structure, function and coronary circulation; technically demanding
Peripheral circulation		
Upper limb cuff occlusion followed by sudden release of occlusion	Ultrasound Doppler	Also known as *brachial artery flow-mediated dilatation*- the current 'gold-standard' for non-invasive assessment of endothelial function; reproducibility major issue
Upper limb cuff occlusion followed by sudden release of occlusion	Digital pulse amplitude tonometry	Emerging as a promising alternative to brachial artery flow-mediated dilatation
Upper limb cuff occlusion followed by sudden release of occlusion	Magnetic resonance imaging	Expensive, limited availability
Inhaled salbutamol and other vasoactive substances	• Pulse wave analysis by applanation tonometry • Pulse contour analysis by digital plethysmography • Laser Doppler skin flowmetry	Technical difficulties; presently used mainly for research purposes
Brachial artery acetylcholine injection	Ultrasound Doppler	Invasive, not suitable for routine clinical application
Brachial artery acetylcholine injection	Strain gauge plethysmography	Invasive, not suitable for routine clinical application

Non-Invasive Evaluation of CBF Response (Table 1)

Given the invasive nature of conventional methods of coronary endothelial function assessment, several non-invasive methods have been tried for this purpose, such as cardiac MRI, PET scan, CBF measurement on Doppler echocardiography and myocardial contrast echocardiography. Among them, cardiac MRI appears to be the most promising modality.

Cardiac MRI

Cardiac MRI with gadolinium as a flow tracer for measurement of CBF response to intravenous dipyridamole or adenosine infusion is possibly the most promising method for non-invasive assessment of coronary MVD. It is completely non-invasive, free of radiation and allows comprehensive assessment of myocardial blood flow whether the perfusion defect is segmental or global and whether it is subendocardial or subepicardial [21,72]. Previous studies with cardiac MRI and invasive assessment of coronary MVD have shown good correlation between the two techniques [73]. The WISE Ancillary Study is currently underway to determine the exact value of cardiac MRI in diagnosis and prognostication of women with CSX [74].

Cardiac MR spectroscopy can also detect stress induced abnormalities of phosphorus metabolism as the metabolic marker of ischemia [16]. However, this technique is limited by the cost and by its inability to explore beyond the anterior wall of the heart.

PET Scan

PET scan helps in measuring average CBF per gram of myocardial tissue and therefore can be applied to identify coronary MVD in the same manner as cardiac MRI [20]. However, the studies using PET scan have so far shown inconsistent findings [75,76].

CBF Measurement on Transthoracic Doppler Echocardiography

CBF in the left anterior descending (LAD) artery can be measured by Doppler echocardiography and its response to intravenous adenosine or dipyridamole can be determined. Because it is completely non-invasive and is readily available, it can be used as the first non-invasive method to identify coronary MVD in patients with suspected CSX [72,77]. In a study by Lanza et al, good correlation was found between Doppler echocardiography based assessment of CBF response in LAD and the cardiac MRI findings [72]. However, the test has limited sensitivity in presence of mild coronary MVD and can be applied only for the LAD. In addition, it is highly dependent on image quality and can be technically very difficult in patients with limited acoustic window.

Myocardial Contrast Echocardiography

Myocardial contrast echocardiography is a relatively new technique that allows both qualitative and quantitative assessment of myocardial perfusion. The currently used ultrasound contrast agents are solutions of microbubbles which are composed of a thin lipid shell filled with an inner core of an inert fluorocarbon gas. When injected intravenously, these microbubbles traverse the pulmonary circulation and reach the left heart and subsequently coronary microcirculation.

Contrast-specific imaging protocols are available that allow visualization of these bubbles within the left ventricular myocardium, permit quantitation of total myocardial blood volume and also allow assessment of myocardial blood flow kinetics. When combined with exercise or pharmacological stressor, this technique can be used for detection of inducible myocardial ischemia with good level of accuracy, as shown in the studies in patients with obstructive CAD [78-80].

Recently, a study by Galiuto and Lanza confirmed the accuracy of myocardial contrast echocardiography for assessment of coronary flow reserve in patients with CSX also [77]. However, more work is needed before it can be routinely recommended for this purpose.

Surrogate Tests (Table 1)

It is now well known that the vascular injury resulting from various atherosclerotic risk factors is a global phenomenon, affecting all the vascular beds sooner or later. Based on this premise, several diagnostic techniques have been developed that, by assessing structure and function of the peripheral vessels, provide indirect information about the state of the coronary arteries and the overall CV risk.

The most extensively evaluated among them are carotid intima-media thickness, brachial artery flow mediated dilatation (BAFMD) and pulse wave velocity. Of these, BAFMD specifically evaluates vascular endothelial function. Since endothelial dysfunction is considered to play a vital role in the pathogenesis of CSX, BAFMD has been studied in CSX patients also. Initial studies have shown high prevalence of impaired BAFMD in these patients, confirming the generalized nature of endothelial dysfunction [35,36]. However, the diagnostic and therapeutic implications of such a finding and consequently, the clinical utility of this test in patients with CSX are yet to be determined.

There are several other non-invasive tests available for assessment of endothelial function in peripheral circulation such as digital pulse amplitude tonometry, laser Doppler skin flowmetry, etc [27,81]. However, their role in patients with CSX has not been fully explored.

Therapeutic Approach

Much like the diagnostic work-up of the patients with CSX, their treatment is also quite challenging. In most patients, no single underlying pathogenic mechanism is identifiable, which makes selection of the appropriate therapeutic agent difficult. Moreover, no therapeutic agent is currently available that can effectively correct the commonly encountered pathological abnormalities- MVD, endothelial dysfunction and abnormal pain perception- in these patients. Accordingly, sub-optimal therapeutic response is common with many patients continuing to have recurrent episodes of chest pain, resulting in significant amount of morbidity. Both the treating physician and the patient need to be fully aware of this so that they are prepared to face and overcome the challenges encountered during this process.

The treatment of CSX usually has a multipronged approach (figure 4). The major components of the therapeutic approach include- 1) aggressive lifestyle changes for the control of CV risk factors, 2) antianginal treatment, 3) correction of MVD/ endothelial dysfunction, 4) analgesic agents, and 5) psychological intervention. While the lifestyle changes and risk factor management are integral components of any therapeutic strategy, the relative emphasis on other components needs to be individualized. Every effort must be made to identify the most likely pathogenic mechanism responsible for the symptoms in a given patient and the therapy should then be tailored accordingly.

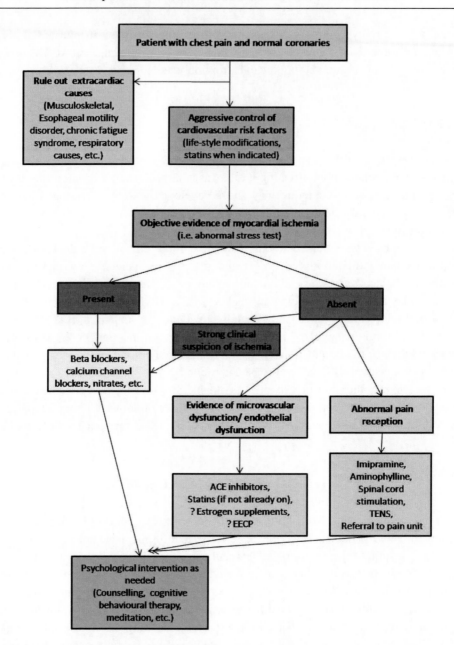

Figure 4. Practical algorithm for management of patients with cardiac syndrome X. ACE- angiotensin-converting enzyme; EECP- enhanced external counterpulsation; TENS- transcutaneous electrical nerve stimulation..

Life Style Changes

Life style changes such as increased physical activity, weight reduction, dietary modifications and smoking cessation play a very important role in the management of CSX [6,82]. All these measures are known to improve the CV health and reduce the risk of adverse cardiac events through multiple beneficial mechanisms [83]. In particular, they all, directly or indirectly, improve endothelial dysfunction, which is a key pathological abnormality in patients with CSX.

In addition, as CSX patients are usually physically deconditioned, have an impaired exercise capacity and have low pain threshold, regular physical training has been shown to improve the pain threshold and reduce the frequency and the severity of angina episodes in them [84].

Antianginal Agents

Given the central role played by myocardial ischemia in causation of symptoms in patients with CSX, all the conventional and non-conventional antianginal drugs (β-blockers, calcium channel blockers, nitrates, K^+ channel openers, trimetazidine, ranolazine, etc) have been tried in these patients. Among them, the β-blockers (atenolol has been tested the most) appear to be the most effective and have most consistently shown benefit in the trials conducted so far [5,85-87]. They reduce the frequency and the severity of angina episodes and improve the exercise duration and the overall quality of life in these patients. Lanza et al studied the effects of atenolol, amlodipine and isosorbide-5-mononitrate on anginal symptoms in 10 patients with CSX in a double-blind, crossover, randomized trial. Among the three agents, only atenolol was found to significantly improve chest pain episodes [85]. Similarly, Bugiardini et al compared propranolol and verapamil in 16 patients with CSX, using Holter monitoring. As compared to verapamil, propranolol was found to be much more effective in reducing the frequency of ischemic episodes in these patients [86].

Calcium channel blockers (nifedipine, diltiazem, nisoldipine, amlodipine, etc) are the other class of drugs that have shown benefit but the results have been less consistent [88,89]. The role of nitrates in the treatment of CSX is uncertain. While the observational studies have suggested that the nitrate use is effective in controlling symptoms in 40–50% of CSX patients others have reported worsening of symptoms with nitrates [59,64,90,91]. Similarly, the role of other antianginal agents such as nikorandil (a K^+ channel opener), trimetazidine, etc. is also not yet clear [88].

The patient subset most likely to benefit with antianginal therapy is the one in which there is strong suggestion of myocardial ischemia as the underlying cause of symptoms. In such patients, therapy with one of the cardio-selective β-blockers should be initiated at the outset itself, provided there is no contraindication to their use. In patients with contraindications to β-blockers, calcium-channel blockers appear to be a reasonable alternative.

Treatment Targeted at Correction of MVD and Endothelial Dysfunction

Statins

Statins are among the most powerful pharmacological agents currently available for the reduction of CV events. Among all the currently available lipid lowering agents, they have the most potent low density lipoprotein cholesterol lowering effect. More importantly, statins also produce multiple beneficial effects beyond just cholesterol lowering such as improvement in endothelial function, anti-inflammatory effects, plaque stabilization, antioxidant effects, etc. Through both these lipid-lowering and non lipid-lowering mechanisms, statins significantly reduce the risk of CV events in a range of cardiac conditions including stable CAD, acute coronary syndromes, aortic stenosis, atrial fibrillation, etc. as well as in a number of non-cardiac illnesses [83,92-95].

Owing to their effect on the endothelial function, statins have been tried in CSX also. In a randomized, prospective study on 40 patients with CSX, pravastatin (40 mg/day) for 3 months was compared with a placebo. After the treatment, BAFMD improved significantly in the pravastatin group- an effect which was accompanied by a significant reduction in the ischemic symptoms. In a quarter of these patients, the ischemic symptoms and the ECG changes during exercise test disappeared completely while no such effects were noted in the placebo group [46]. Similar findings have been reported by many other investigators also [96].

Angiotensin-Converting Enzyme Inhibitors

Similar to statins, angiotensin-converting enzyme (ACE) inhibitors also have a number of beneficial effects on the vascular system with improvement in the endothelial function being one of them. In addition, ACE inhibitors also attenuate sympathetic system activity resulting in systemic vasodilatation. It has been proposed that this vasodilatory effect may be an important mechanism responsible for reduction of exercise-induced ischemia seen with ACE-inhibitors in patients with CSX [97,98].

Estrogen Therapy

As mentioned above, given the high prevalence of postmenopausal women in the CSX patient populations, estrogen deficiency has been considered to play a causative role. Accordingly, hormone replacement therapy has drawn considerable attention as a treatment option for women with CSX. However, the studies conducted with different hormone preparations so far have shown conflicting results [43,99-101] while some have demonstrated reduced angina frequency and severity, others have shown little or no symptomatic effect at all. On the other hand, many large-scale trials in postmenopausal women have clearly shown an increased risk of cardiac events and breast cancer with different types of hormone supplements [102-104]. Therefore, in view of the lack of a definite symptomatic benefit and unequivocal risk of harm, the use of hormone-replacement therapy as a treatment for CSX should be discouraged. However, estrogen supplements can be tried in a small proportion of CSX patients in whom a direct relationship can be demonstrated between estrogen deficiency and the symptoms. In such cases, it is advisable to educate the patient about the potential risks and to involve her in the decision-making.

Enhanced External Counterpulsation

Enhanced external counterpulsation (EECP) has emerged as a therapeutic option for CAD patients who have significant ischemic symptoms but their disease is not amenable to revascularization due to some reason. The proposed mechanisms believed to underlie the beneficial effects of EECP include improvement in endothelial function, promotion of collateralization, ventricular function enhancement, and peripheral effects resembling those seen with regular physical exercise [105]. In view of the potential effects of EECP on endothelial function, it has been tried in patients with CSX also. In a few studies, EECP has been shown to result in significant symptomatic improvement in CSX patients presenting with severe angina refractory to the pharmacological treatment [106]. Moreover, the benefit has been shown to persist for several months after the initial course of treatment [107].

Analgesic Agents

A number of analgesic interventions have been tried in patients with CSX with variable results. Imipramine, an antidepressant with analgesic properties, has been evaluated the most for this purpose. Numerous studies have shown it reduces symptoms in patients with CSX, though its effect on overall quality of life has been questioned by some [108,109]. Similarly, benzodiazepines such as diazepam have also been tried due to their analgesic, anti-inflammatory and muscle relaxant effects and have been reported to improve symptoms [110]. Xanthine derivatives, such as aminophylline, have also been shown to produce symptomatic benefit in patients with CSX through inhibition of the adenosine receptors [111,112].

In patients refractory to the conventional treatment, non-pharmacological measures such as transcutaneous electrical nerve stimulation and spinal cord stimulation can be tried [113-115]. Spinal cord stimulation, in particular, has been shown to result in significant improvement in symptoms through alteration of coronary microvascular tone and also through modification of the pain-handling pathways [115].

Psychological Intervention

Since psychological disturbances are commonly encountered in patients with CSX, different forms of psychological therapies have been employed with variable success in the management of CSX. Patient counselling, structured cognitive behavioural therapy, meditation, etc have all been shown to produce benefit [116-118]. These measures can reduce the frequency of angina, improve quality of life and can also ameliorate exercise induced ST-T changes. The treatment is more likely to be successful if it is initiated early after the diagnosis.

Prognosis

Most of the earlier studies had suggested a benign prognosis for patients with CSX with the incidence of major adverse cardiac events being similar to that observed in age and sex matched healthy controls [59]. However, more recent studies have shown that the prognosis in these patients may not necessarily be as benign as previously reported [119-123]. This is particularly true for the patients who have evidence of MVD or endothelial dysfunction [124,125]. The WISE study clearly showed that the patients with CSX who also had evidence of microcirculatory dysfunction, frequently had subclinical atherosclerosis on intravascular ultrasound and were at appreciable risk (as high as 2.5% per year) of adverse cardiac events.

In another recent report, which included nearly 5200 patients with normal coronary arteries or diffuse non-obstructive CAD, the risk of major adverse cardiac events and all-cause mortality was found to be elevated in them, as compared to the reference population [123]. Similar findings have been reported in other studies as well [121,122]. Nonetheless, the overall adverse risk in patients with CSX is still much lower than that observed in patients presenting with same symptoms but also having obstructive CAD. Similarly, development of left ventricular systolic dysfunction is also rare in these patients [59].

Although the mortality in patients with CSX may not be high, the condition results in a huge amount of morbidity and therefore, remains a major healthcare challenge. The quality of life is significantly compromised in a large proportion of patients due to repeated episodes of chest pain which may result in considerable restriction of daily activities. The lack of adequate relief from the symptoms leads to considerable anxiety, disrupts personal life and also adversely affects the family. Furthermore, the persistence of symptoms may lead to frequent hospitalisation for diagnostic and therapeutic purposes resulting in frequent absence from work and the consequent loss of productivity.

References

[1]   Kemp HG, Kronmal RA, Vlietstra RE, Frye RL. Seven year survival of patients with normal or near normal coronary arteriograms: a CASS registry study. *J Am Coll Cardiol* 1986;7:479-83.

[2]   Sharaf BL, Pepine CJ, Kerensky RA, Reis SE, Reichek N, Rogers WJ, et al. Detailed angiographic analysis of women with suspected ischemic chest pain (pilot phase data from the NHLBI-sponsored Women's Ischemia Syndrome Evaluation [WISE] Study Angiographic Core Laboratory). *Am J Cardiol* 2001;87:937-41; A3.

[3]   Proudfit WL, Shirey EK, Sones FM, Jr. Selective cine coronary arteriography. Correlation with clinical findings in 1,000 patients. *Circulation* 1966;33:901-10.

[4]   Kemp HG, Jr. Left ventricular function in patients with the anginal syndrome and normal coronary arteriograms. *Am J Cardiol* 1973;32:375-6.

[5]   Lanza GA. Cardiac syndrome X: a critical overview and future perspectives. *Heart* 2007;93:159-66.

[6]   Kaski JC. Pathophysiology and management of patients with chest pain and normal coronary arteriograms (cardiac syndrome X). *Circulation* 2004;109:568-72.

[7]   Cannon RO, 3rd. Microvascular angina and the continuing dilemma of chest pain with normal coronary angiograms. *J Am Coll Cardiol* 2009;54:877-85.

[8]   Cannon RO, 3rd, Quyyumi AA, Schenke WH, Fananapazir L, Tucker EE, Gaughan AM, et al. Abnormal cardiac sensitivity in patients with chest pain and normal coronary arteries. *J Am Coll Cardiol* 1990;16:1359-66.

[9]   Lagerqvist B, Sylven C, Waldenstrom A. Lower threshold for adenosine-induced chest pain in patients with angina and normal coronary angiograms. *Br Heart J* 1992;68:282-5.

[10]   Cosin-Sales J, Pizzi C, Brown S, Kaski JC. C-reactive protein, clinical presentation, and ischemic activity in patients with chest pain and normal coronary angiograms. *J Am Coll Cardiol* 2003;41:1468-74.

[11] Guzik P, Rogacka D, Trachalski J, Minczykowski A, Balinski M, Wykretowicz A, et al. Comparison of the exercise treadmill test and 24-hour ECG Holter monitoring in patients with syndrome X or coronary atherosclerosis. *Kardiol Pol* 2007;65:262-9; discussion 270-1.

[12] Ruggeri A, Taruschio G, Loricchio ML, Samory G, Borghi A, Bugiardini R. [The correlation between the clinical characteristics and psychological status in syndrome X patients]. *Cardiologia* 1996;41:551-7.

[13] Tweddel AC, Martin W, Hutton I. Thallium scans in syndrome X. *Br Heart J* 1992;68:48-50.

[14] Crea F, Lanza GA. Angina pectoris and normal coronary arteries: cardiac syndrome X. *Heart* 2004;90:457-63.

[15] Buffon A, Rigattieri S, Santini SA, Ramazzotti V, Crea F, Giardina B, et al. Myocardial ischemia-reperfusion damage after pacing-induced tachycardia in patients with cardiac syndrome X. *Am J Physiol Heart Circ Physiol* 2000;279:H2627-33.

[16] Buchthal SD, den Hollander JA, Merz CN, Rogers WJ, Pepine CJ, Reichek N, et al. Abnormal myocardial phosphorus-31 nuclear magnetic resonance spectroscopy in women with chest pain but normal coronary angiograms. *N Engl J Med* 2000;342:829-35.

[17] Nihoyannopoulos P, Kaski JC, Crake T, Maseri A. Absence of myocardial dysfunction during stress in patients with syndrome X. *J Am Coll Cardiol* 1991;18:1463-70.

[18] Panza JA, Laurienzo JM, Curiel RV, Unger EF, Quyyumi AA, Dilsizian V, et al. Investigation of the mechanism of chest pain in patients with angiographically normal coronary arteries using transesophageal dobutamine stress echocardiography. *J Am Coll Cardiol* 1997;29:293-301.

[19] Maseri A, Crea F, Kaski JC, Crake T. Mechanisms of angina pectoris in syndrome X. *J Am Coll Cardiol* 1991;17:499-506.

[20] Bottcher M, Botker HE, Sonne H, Nielsen TT, Czernin J. Endothelium-dependent and -independent perfusion reserve and the effect of L-arginine on myocardial perfusion in patients with syndrome X. *Circulation* 1999;99:1795-801.

[21] Panting JR, Gatehouse PD, Yang GZ, Grothues F, Firmin DN, Collins P, et al. Abnormal subendocardial perfusion in cardiac syndrome X detected by cardiovascular magnetic resonance imaging. *N Engl J Med* 2002;346:1948-53.

[22] Opherk D, Zebe H, Weihe E, Mall G, Durr C, Gravert B, et al. Reduced coronary dilatory capacity and ultrastructural changes of the myocardium in patients with angina pectoris but normal coronary arteriograms. *Circulation* 1981;63:817-25.

[23] Reis SE, Holubkov R, Conrad Smith AJ, Kelsey SF, Sharaf BL, Reichek N, et al. Coronary microvascular dysfunction is highly prevalent in women with chest pain in the absence of coronary artery disease: results from the NHLBI WISE study. *Am Heart J* 2001;141:735-41.

[24] Motz W, Vogt M, Rabenau O, Scheler S, Luckhoff A, Strauer BE. Evidence of endothelial dysfunction in coronary resistance vessels in patients with angina pectoris and normal coronary angiograms. *Am J Cardiol* 1991;68:996-1003.

[25] Egashira K, Inou T, Hirooka Y, Yamada A, Urabe Y, Takeshita A. Evidence of impaired endothelium-dependent coronary vasodilatation in patients with angina pectoris and normal coronary angiograms. *N Engl J Med* 1993;328:1659-64.

[26] Cannon RO, 3rd, Watson RM, Rosing DR, Epstein SE. Angina caused by reduced vasodilator reserve of the small coronary arteries. *J Am Coll Cardiol* 1983;1:1359-73.

[27] Deanfield JE, Halcox JP, Rabelink TJ. Endothelial function and dysfunction: testing and clinical relevance. *Circulation* 2007;115:1285-95.

[28] Martin BJ, Anderson TJ. Risk prediction in cardiovascular disease: the prognostic significance of endothelial dysfunction. *Can J Cardiol* 2009;25 Suppl A:15A-20A.

[29] Furchgott RF, Zawadzki JV. The obligatory role of endothelial cells in the relaxation of arterial smooth muscle by acetylcholine. *Nature* 1980;288:373-6.

[30] Taddei S, Ghiadoni L, Virdis A, Versari D, Salvetti A. Mechanisms of endothelial dysfunction: clinical significance and preventive non-pharmacological therapeutic strategies. *Curr Pharm Des* 2003;9:2385-402.

[31] Zeiher AM, Krause T, Schachinger V, Minners J, Moser E. Impaired endothelium-dependent vasodilation of coronary resistance vessels is associated with exercise-induced myocardial ischemia. *Circulation* 1995;91:2345-52.

[32] Kaski JC, Cox ID, Crook JR, Salomone OA, Fredericks S, Hann C, et al. Differential plasma endothelin levels in subgroups of patients with angina and angiographically normal coronary arteries. Coronary Artery Disease Research Group. *Am Heart J* 1998;136:412-7.

[33] Cox ID, Botker HE, Bagger JP, Sonne HS, Kristensen BO, Kaski JC. Elevated endothelin concentrations are associated with reduced coronary vasomotor responses in patients with chest pain and normal coronary arteriograms. *J Am Coll Cardiol* 1999;34:455-60.

[34] Egashira K, Hirooka Y, Kuga T, Mohri M, Takeshita A. Effects of L-arginine supplementation on endothelium-dependent coronary vasodilation in patients with angina pectoris and normal coronary arteriograms. *Circulation* 1996;94:130-4.

[35] Sax FL, Cannon RO, 3rd, Hanson C, Epstein SE. Impaired forearm vasodilator reserve in patients with microvascular angina. Evidence of a generalized disorder of vascular function? *N Engl J Med* 1987;317:1366-70.

[36] Masci PG, Laclaustra M, Lara JG, Kaski JC. Brachial artery flow-mediated dilation and myocardial perfusion in patients with cardiac syndrome X. *Am J Cardiol* 2005;95:1478-80.

[37] Botker HE, Moller N, Ovesen P, Mengel A, Schmitz O, Orskov H, et al. Insulin resistance in microvascular angina (syndrome X). *Lancet* 1993;342:136-40.

[38] Piatti P, Fragasso G, Monti LD, Caumo A, Van Phan C, Valsecchi G, et al. Endothelial and metabolic characteristics of patients with angina and angiographically normal coronary arteries: comparison with subjects with insulin resistance syndrome and normal controls. *J Am Coll Cardiol* 1999;34:1452-60.

[39] Jadhav S, Ferrell W, Greer IA, Petrie JR, Cobbe SM, Sattar N. Effects of metformin on microvascular function and exercise tolerance in women with angina and normal coronary arteries: a randomized, double-blind, placebo-controlled study. *J Am Coll Cardiol* 2006;48:956-63.

[40] Kaski JC. Overview of gender aspects of cardiac syndrome X. *Cardiovasc Res* 2002;53:620-6.

[41] Roque M, Heras M, Roig E, Masotti M, Rigol M, Betriu A, et al. Short-term effects of transdermal estrogen replacement therapy on coronary vascular reactivity in

postmenopausal women with angina pectoris and normal results on coronary angiograms. *J Am Coll Cardiol* 1998;31:139-43.

[42] Albertsson PA, Emanuelsson H, Milsom I. Beneficial effect of treatment with transdermal estradiol-17-beta on exercise-induced angina and ST segment depression in syndrome X. *Int J Cardiol* 1996;54:13-20.

[43] Rosano GM, Peters NS, Lefroy D, Lindsay DC, Sarrel PM, Collins P, et al. 17-beta-Estradiol therapy lessens angina in postmenopausal women with syndrome X. *J Am Coll Cardiol* 1996;28:1500-5.

[44] Ross R. Atherosclerosis--an inflammatory disease. *N Engl J Med* 1999;340:115-26.

[45] Teragawa H, Fukuda Y, Matsuda K, Ueda K, Higashi Y, Oshima T, et al. Relation between C reactive protein concentrations and coronary microvascular endothelial function. *Heart* 2004;90:750-4.

[46] Arroyo-Espliguero R, Mollichelli N, Avanzas P, Zouridakis E, Newey VR, Nassiri DK, et al. Chronic inflammation and increased arterial stiffness in patients with cardiac syndrome X. *Eur Heart J* 2003;24:2006-11.

[47] Lanza GA, Giordano A, Pristipino C, Calcagni ML, Meduri G, Trani C, et al. Abnormal cardiac adrenergic nerve function in patients with syndrome X detected by [123I]metaiodobenzylguanidine myocardial scintigraphy. *Circulation* 1997;96:821-6.

[48] Lee BK, Durairaj A, Mehra A, Wenby RB, Meiselman HJ, Alexy T. Microcirculatory dysfunction in cardiac syndrome X: role of abnormal blood rheology. *Microcirculation* 2008;15:451-9.

[49] Gaspardone A, Ferri C, Crea F, Versaci F, Tomai F, Santucci A, et al. Enhanced activity of sodium-lithium countertransport in patients with cardiac syndrome X: a potential link between cardiac and metabolic syndrome X. *J Am Coll Cardiol* 1998;32:2031-4.

[50] Shapiro LM, Crake T, Poole-Wilson PA. Is altered cardiac sensation responsible for chest pain in patients with normal coronary arteries? Clinical observation during cardiac catheterisation. *Br Med J* (Clin Res Ed) 1988;296:170-1.

[51] Pasceri V, Lanza GA, Buffon A, Montenero AS, Crea F, Maseri A. Role of abnormal pain sensitivity and behavioral factors in determining chest pain in syndrome X. *J Am Coll Cardiol* 1998;31:62-6.

[52] Turiel M, Galassi AR, Glazier JJ, Kaski JC, Maseri A. Pain threshold and tolerance in women with syndrome X and women with stable angina pectoris. *Am J Cardiol* 1987;60:503-7.

[53] Cannon RO, 3rd, Cattau EL, Jr., Yakshe PN, Maher K, Schenke WH, Benjamin SB, et al. Coronary flow reserve, esophageal motility, and chest pain in patients with angiographically normal coronary arteries. *Am J Med* 1990;88:217-22.

[54] Rosen SD, Paulesu E, Wise RJ, Camici PG. Central neural contribution to the perception of chest pain in cardiac syndrome X. *Heart* 2002;87:513-9.

[55] Rosen SD, Paulesu E, Frith CD, Frackowiak RS, Davies GJ, Jones T, et al. Central nervous pathways mediating angina pectoris. *Lancet* 1994;344:147-50.

[56] Lanza GA, Sestito A, Sgueglia GA, Infusino F, Papacci F, Visocchi M, et al. Effect of spinal cord stimulation on spontaneous and stress-induced angina and 'ischemia-like' ST-segment depression in patients with cardiac syndrome X. *Eur Heart J* 2005;26:983-9.

[57]   Lanza GA. Abnormal cardiac nerve function in syndrome X. *Herz* 1999;24:97-106.

[58]   Fedele F, Agati L, Pugliese M, Cervellini P, Benedetti G, Magni G, et al. Role of the central endogenous opiate system in patients with syndrome X. *Am Heart J* 1998;136:1003-9.

[59]   Kaski JC, Rosano GM, Collins P, Nihoyannopoulos P, Maseri A, Poole-Wilson PA. Cardiac syndrome X: clinical characteristics and left ventricular function. Long-term follow-up study. *J Am Coll Cardiol* 1995;25:807-14.

[60]   Beitman BD, Mukerji V, Lamberti JW, Schmid L, DeRosear L, Kushner M, et al. Panic disorder in patients with chest pain and angiographically normal coronary arteries. *Am J Cardiol* 1989;63:1399-403.

[61]   Rosen SD. Hearts and minds: psychological factors and the chest pain of cardiac syndrome X. *Eur Heart J* 2004;25:1672-4.

[62]   Rosen SD, Corlando AP, Camici PG. Psychological assessment of syndrome X patients. *Br Heart J* 1994;71:P23.

[63]   Pupita G, Kaski JC, Galassi AR, Gavrielides S, Crea F, Maseri A. Similar time course of ST depression during and after exercise in patients with coronary artery disease and syndrome X. *Am Heart J* 1990;120:848-54.

[64]   Lanza GA, Manzoli A, Bia E, Crea F, Maseri A. Acute effects of nitrates on exercise testing in patients with syndrome X. Clinical and pathophysiological implications. *Circulation* 1994;90:2695-700.

[65]   Meller J, Goldsmith SJ, Rudin A, Pichard AD, Gorlin R, Teichholz LE, et al. Spectrum of exercise thallium-201 myocardial perfusion imaging in patients with chest pain and normal coronary angiograms. *Am J Cardiol* 1979;43:717-23.

[66]   Berger BC, Abramowitz R, Park CH, Desai AG, Madsen MT, Chung EK, et al. Abnormal thallium-201 scans in patients with chest pain and angiographically normal coronary arteries. *Am J Cardiol* 1983;52:365-70.

[67]   Dunn RF, Wolff L, Wagner S, Botvinick EH. The inconsistent pattern of thallium defects: a clue to the false positive perfusion scintigram. *Am J Cardiol* 1981;48:224-32.

[68]   Brown KA, Osbakken M, Boucher CA, Strauss HW, Pohost GM, Okada RD. Positive exercise thallium-201 test responses in patients with less than 50% maximal coronary stenosis: angiographic and clinical predictors. *Am J Cardiol* 1985;55:54-7.

[69]   Kaul S, Newell JB, Chesler DA, Pohost GM, Okada RD, Boucher CA. Quantitative thallium imaging findings in patients with normal coronary angiographic findings and in clinically normal subjects. *Am J Cardiol* 1986;57:509-12.

[70]   Rosano GM, Peters NS, Kaski JC, Mavrogeni SI, Collins P, Underwood RS, et al. Abnormal uptake and washout of thallium-201 in patients with syndrome X and normal-appearing scans. *Am J Cardiol* 1995;75:400-2.

[71]   Pries AR, Habazettl H, Ambrosio G, Hansen PR, Kaski JC, Schachinger V, et al. A review of methods for assessment of coronary microvascular disease in both clinical and experimental settings. *Cardiovasc Res* 2008;80:165-74.

[72]   Lanza GA, Buffon A, Sestito A, Natale L, Sgueglia GA, Galiuto L, et al. Relation between stress-induced myocardial perfusion defects on cardiovascular magnetic resonance and coronary microvascular dysfunction in patients with cardiac syndrome X. *J Am Coll Cardiol* 2008;51:466-72.

[73] Wohrle J, Nusser T, Merkle N, Kestler HA, Grebe OC, Marx N, et al. Myocardial perfusion reserve in cardiovascular magnetic resonance: Correlation to coronary microvascular dysfunction. *J Cardiovasc Magn Reson* 2006;8:781-7.

[74] Shufelt C, Kar S, Slivka M, Thomson L, Yang Y, Berman D, et al. Cardiac magnetic resonance imaging and coronary reactivity testing: a useful noninvasive tool. *J Am Coll Cardiol* 2008;51:A231.

[75] Galassi AR, Crea F, Araujo LI, Lammertsma AA, Pupita G, Yamamoto Y, et al. Comparison of regional myocardial blood flow in syndrome X and one-vessel coronary artery disease. *Am J Cardiol* 1993;72:134-9.

[76] Geltman EM, Henes CG, Senneff MJ, Sobel BE, Bergmann SR. Increased myocardial perfusion at rest and diminished perfusion reserve in patients with angina and angiographically normal coronary arteries. *J Am Coll Cardiol* 1990;16:586-95.

[77] Galiuto L, Sestito A, Barchetta S, Sgueglia GA, Infusino F, La Rosa C, et al. Noninvasive evaluation of flow reserve in the left anterior descending coronary artery in patients with cardiac syndrome X. *Am J Cardiol* 2007;99:1378-83.

[78] Kaul S, Senior R, Dittrich H, Raval U, Khattar R, Lahiri A. Detection of coronary artery disease with myocardial contrast echocardiography: comparison with 99mTc-sestamibi single-photon emission computed tomography. *Circulation* 1997;96:785-92.

[79] Moir S, Haluska BA, Jenkins C, Fathi R, Marwick TH. Incremental benefit of myocardial contrast to combined dipyridamole-exercise stress echocardiography for the assessment of coronary artery disease. *Circulation* 2004;110:1108-13.

[80] Dijkmans PA, Senior R, Becher H, Porter TR, Wei K, Visser CA, et al. Myocardial contrast echocardiography evolving as a clinically feasible technique for accurate, rapid, and safe assessment of myocardial perfusion: the evidence so far. *J Am Coll Cardiol* 2006;48:2168-77.

[81] Al-Qaisi M, Kharbanda RK, Mittal TK, Donald AE. Measurement of endothelial function and its clinical utility for cardiovascular risk. *Vasc Health Risk Manag* 2008;4:647-52.

[82] Mehta PK, Bairey Merz CN. Treatment of angina in subjects with evidence of myocardial ischemia and no obstructive coronary artery disease. In: Bonow RO, ed. *Braunwald's Heart Disease*. 9th ed. Philadelphia, PA: Elsevier, 2011.

[83] Executive Summary of The Third Report of The National Cholesterol Education Program (NCEP) Expert Panel on Detection, Evaluation, And Treatment of High Blood Cholesterol In Adults (Adult Treatment Panel III). *Jama* 2001;285:2486-97.

[84] Eriksson BE, Tyni-Lenne R, Svedenhag J, Hallin R, Jensen-Urstad K, Jensen-Urstad M, et al. Physical training in Syndrome X: physical training counteracts deconditioning and pain in Syndrome X. *J Am Coll Cardiol* 2000;36:1619-25.

[85] Lanza GA, Colonna G, Pasceri V, Maseri A. Atenolol versus amlodipine versus isosorbide-5-mononitrate on anginal symptoms in syndrome X. *Am J Cardiol* 1999;84:854-6, A8.

[86] Bugiardini R, Borghi A, Biagetti L, Puddu P. Comparison of verapamil versus propranolol therapy in syndrome X. *Am J Cardiol* 1989;63:286-90.

[87] Bairey Merz CN, Pepine CJ. Syndrome X and microvascular coronary dysfunction. *Circulation* 2011;124:1477-80.

[88] Kaski JC, Valenzuela Garcia LF. Therapeutic options for the management of patients with cardiac syndrome X. *Eur Heart J* 2001;22:283-93.

[89] Ozcelik F, Altun A, Ozbay G. Antianginal and anti-ischemic effects of nisoldipine and ramipril in patients with syndrome X. *Clin Cardiol* 1999;22:361-5.

[90] Radice M, Giudici V, Albertini A, Mannarini A. Usefulness of changes in exercise tolerance induced by nitroglycerin in identifying patients with syndrome X. *Am Heart J* 1994;127:531-5.

[91] Radice M, Giudici V, Pusineri E, Breghi L, Nicoli T, Peci P, et al. Different effects of acute administration of aminophylline and nitroglycerin on exercise capacity in patients with syndrome X. *Am J Cardiol* 1996;78:88-92.

[92] Davignon J. Beneficial cardiovascular pleiotropic effects of statins. *Circulation* 2004;109:III39-43.

[93] Baigent C, Landray M, Warren M. Statin therapy in kidney disease populations: potential benefits beyond lipid lowering and the need for clinical trials. *Curr Opin Nephrol Hypertens* 2004;13:601-5.

[94] Young RP, Hopkins R, Eaton TE. Potential benefits of statins on morbidity and mortality in chronic obstructive pulmonary disease: a review of the evidence. *Postgrad Med J* 2009;85:414-21.

[95] Marzilli M. Pleiotropic effects of statins: evidence for benefits beyond LDL-cholesterol lowering. *Am J Cardiovasc Drugs* 2010;10 Suppl 1:3-9.

[96] Kayikcioglu M, Payzin S, Yavuzgil O, Kultursay H, Can LH, Soydan I. Benefits of statin treatment in cardiac syndrome-X. *Eur Heart J* 2003;24:1999-2005.

[97] Kaski JC, Rosano G, Gavrielides S, Chen L. Effects of angiotensin-converting enzyme inhibition on exercise-induced angina and ST segment depression in patients with microvascular angina. *J Am Coll Cardiol* 1994;23:652-7.

[98] Nalbantgil I, Onder R, Altintig A, Nalbantgil S, Kiliccioglu B, Boydak B, et al. Therapeutic benefits of cilazapril in patients with syndrome X. *Cardiology* 1998;89:130-3.

[99] Lee TM, Su SF, Lee YT, Tsai CH. Effect of estrogen on ventricular repolarization in menopausal patients with syndrome X and effects of nicorandil. *Am J Cardiol* 1999;84:65-9.

[100] Adamson DL, Webb CM, Collins P. Esterified estrogens combined with methyltestosterone improve emotional well-being in postmenopausal women with chest pain and normal coronary angiograms. *Menopause* 2001;8:233-8.

[101] Sitges M, Heras M, Roig E, Duran M, Masotti M, Zurbano MJ, et al. Acute and mid-term combined hormone replacement therapy improves endothelial function in post-menopausal women with angina and angiographically normal coronary arteries. *Eur Heart J* 2001;22:2116-24.

[102] Beral V. Breast cancer and hormone-replacement therapy in the Million Women Study. *Lancet* 2003;362:419-27.

[103] Hulley S, Grady D, Bush T, Furberg C, Herrington D, Riggs B, et al. Randomized trial of estrogen plus progestin for secondary prevention of coronary heart disease in postmenopausal women. Heart and Estrogen/progestin Replacement Study (HERS) Research Group. *JAMA* 1998;280:605-13.

[104] Paoletti R, Wenger NK. Review of the International Position Paper on Women's Health and Menopause: a comprehensive approach. *Circulation* 2003;107:1336-9.

[105] Manchanda A, Soran O. Enhanced external counterpulsation and future directions: step beyond medical management for patients with angina and heart failure. *J Am Coll Cardiol* 2007;50:1523-31.

[106] Bonetti PO, Gadasalli SN, Lerman A, Barsness GW. Successful treatment of symptomatic coronary endothelial dysfunction with enhanced external counterpulsation. *Mayo Clin Proc* 2004;79:690-2.

[107] Kronhaus KD, Lawson WE. Enhanced external counterpulsation is an effective treatment for Syndrome X. *Int J Cardiol* 2009;135:256-7.

[108] Cannon RO, 3rd, Quyyumi AA, Mincemoyer R, Stine AM, Gracely RH, Smith WB, et al. Imipramine in patients with chest pain despite normal coronary angiograms. *N Engl J Med* 1994;330:1411-7.

[109] Cox ID, Hann CM, Kaski JC. Low dose imipramine improves chest pain but not quality of life in patients with angina and normal coronary angiograms. *Eur Heart J* 1998;19:250-4.

[110] Huffman JC, Stern TA. The use of benzodiazepines in the treatment of chest pain: a review of the literature. *J Emerg Med* 2003;25:427-37.

[111] Elliott PM, Krzyzowska-Dickinson K, Calvino R, Hann C, Kaski JC. Effect of oral aminophylline in patients with angina and normal coronary arteriograms (cardiac syndrome X). *Heart* 1997;77:523-6.

[112] Yoshio H, Shimizu M, Kita Y, Ino H, Kaku B, Taki J, et al. Effects of short-term aminophylline administration on cardiac functional reserve in patients with syndrome X. *J Am Coll Cardiol* 1995;25:1547-51.

[113] Chauhan A, Mullins PA, Thuraisingham SI, Taylor G, Petch MC, Schofield PM. Effect of transcutaneous electrical nerve stimulation on coronary blood flow. *Circulation* 1994;89:694-702.

[114] Sanderson JE, Woo KS, Chung HK, Chan WW, Tse LK, White HD. The effect of transcutaneous electrical nerve stimulation on coronary and systemic haemodynamics in syndrome X. *Coron Artery Dis* 1996;7:547-52.

[115] Lanza GA, Sestito A, Sandric S, Cioni B, Tamburrini G, Barollo A, et al. Spinal cord stimulation in patients with refractory anginal pain and normal coronary arteries. *Ital Heart J* 2001;2:25-30.

[116] Mayou RA, Bryant BM, Sanders D, Bass C, Klimes I, Forfar C. A controlled trial of cognitive behavioural therapy for non-cardiac chest pain. *Psychol Med* 1997;27:1021-31.

[117] Potts SG, Lewin R, Fox KA, Johnstone EC. Group psychological treatment for chest pain with normal coronary arteries. *QJM* 1999;92:81-6.

[118] van Peski-Oosterbaan AS, Spinhoven P, van Rood Y, van der Does JW, Bruschke AV, Rooijmans HG. Cognitive-behavioral therapy for noncardiac chest pain: a randomized trial. *Am J Med* 1999;106:424-9.

[119] Bugiardini R, Bairey Merz CN. Angina with "normal" coronary arteries: a changing philosophy. *JAMA* 2005;293:477-84.

[120] Opherk D, Schuler G, Wetterauer K, Manthey J, Schwarz F, Kubler W. Four-year follow-up study in patients with angina pectoris and normal coronary arteriograms ("syndrome X"). *Circulation* 1989;80:1610-6.

[121] Pepine CJ, Anderson RD, Sharaf BL, Reis SE, Smith KM, Handberg EM, et al. Coronary microvascular reactivity to adenosine predicts adverse outcome in women evaluated for suspected ischemia results from the National Heart, Lung and Blood Institute WISE (Women's Ischemia Syndrome Evaluation) study. *J Am Coll Cardiol* 2010;55:2825-32.

[122] von Mering GO, Arant CB, Wessel TR, McGorray SP, Bairey Merz CN, Sharaf BL, et al. Abnormal coronary vasomotion as a prognostic indicator of cardiovascular events in women: results from the National Heart, Lung, and Blood Institute-Sponsored Women's Ischemia Syndrome Evaluation (WISE). *Circulation* 2004;109:722-5.

[123] Jespersen L, Hvelplund A, Abildstrom SZ, Pedersen F, Galatius S, Madsen JK, et al. Stable angina pectoris with no obstructive coronary artery disease is associated with increased risks of major adverse cardiovascular events. *Eur Heart J* 2012;33:734-44.

[124] Bugiardini R, Manfrini O, Pizzi C, Fontana F, Morgagni G. Endothelial function predicts future development of coronary artery disease: a study of women with chest pain and normal coronary angiograms. *Circulation* 2004;109:2518-23.

[125] Halcox JP, Schenke WH, Zalos G, Mincemoyer R, Prasad A, Waclawiw MA, et al. Prognostic value of coronary vascular endothelial dysfunction. *Circulation* 2002;106:653-8.

In: Current Issues in the Management of Stable Ischemic Heart … ISBN: 978-1-62417-203-8
Editor: Mukesh Singh   © 2013 Nova Science Publishers, Inc.

Chapter VII

Recent Advances in the Pathophysiology and Management of Microvascular Angina

K. S. Sandhu[*]

West Midlands Deanery, UK

Abstract

The syndrome consisting of cardiac sounding chest pain with ischemic changes on electrocardiogram or stress imaging during exertion but no obstructive lesions on diagnostic coronary angiography was first described in 1973, when it was termed syndrome X. It was later changed to microvascular angina on recognition of the pathophysiology originating within the microvascular myocardial blood supply. The pathophysiology was initially attributed solely to be due to ischemia, however more recently microvascular circulation abnormalities, endothelial dysfunction, sympathetic over activity, metabolic derangement, abnormal pain perception, effects of oestrogen, and inflammation have all been implicated. The syndrome effects predominantly females and was historically thought of as being benign, but more recently linked with morbidity and mortality, albeit not as significant when compared to patients with obstructive epicardial disease. No current national or international guidelines exist on how to best manage such patients and therefore a number of suggestions have been made after small trials. Management currently involves rehabilitation, smoking cessation, use of statins, ACE-inhibitors, nitrates, calcium channel blockers, beta blockers, tricyclic antidepressants, spinal cord stimulation and even cognitive behavioural therapy. The combination of a number of possible aetiologies and therefore patient management strategies suggest a complex syndrome. We have progressed over the last 40 years however the exact pathophysiology and most appropriate treatment still eludes us today and therefore further work is still required.

[*] Address for correspondence: Dr K S Sandhu. Specialist Registrar,WestMidlands Deanery,United Kingdom.Email: ksandhu@hotmail.com.

Introduction

The current diagnostic model of chest pain focuses on significant obstructions within the large coronary epicardial arteries as the cause for angina.However, angina in the setting of non-obstructive coronary artery has been recognized for over 40 years [1]. The triad of typical angina chest pain, ST-segment changes suggestive of myocardial ischemia in a patient with completely normal coronary arteriogram was first termed "cardiac syndrome X", by Harvey Kemp in 1973 [2]. Thereafter the term "microvascular angina" was proposed in 1983 [3,4,5]. This was based on reports published in the mid-1980s that suggested significant, albeit, transient constriction of coronary microcirculation that had the potential for severely impairing myocardial perfusion. Thereby causing cardiac ischemia and its associated symptoms. Since this proposal had involvement of smaller vessels as the pathophysiological cause the term microvascular angina (MVA), was coined[4,5,6].

This phenomenon is a common clinical dilemma[7,8]. Many authors note the occurrence of ischemic heart disease in the absence of significant obstructive coronary on angiography with a female bias [9,10,11]. The Coronary Artery Surgery Study (CASS) found that greater than 50% and 17% of females and males respectively that had diagnostic coronary angiography for classical angina like chest pain had non obstructive coronary arteries [8]. In fact 13-30% of patients with electrocardiographic and perfusion imagining demonstrating ischemia hadnon-obstructive epicardial arteries on angiography [12,13,14].Interestingly Sullivan et al found that almost 100% of men but only 59% of women had significant coronary artery disease on angiography [15].Many authors stress that prior to diagnosing normal or near normal angiogram care needs to be taken not to rule out possible hidden lesion and if in doubt to investigate these fully with intravascular ultrasound or calculation of fractional flow reserves [16,17].

There have been a number of studies having tried to categorise symptoms with gender. Nausea, emesis, jaw, neck and back pain [18] SOB indigestion and palpitations [19,20] seemed to be more associated with females. Diaphoresis was more commonly seen in men [18]. Yet other studies have found no gender difference of symptoms [21,22,23]. There has also been a suggestion that gender differences in symptoms may be in part attributed to women being better able to communicate and men considering symptoms as trivial [24].

Once thought of a benign diagnosis it has now largely been accepted that the syndrome carries with it mortality, morbidity and therefore an associated heavy economic burden[25]. The mortality is however less with non-obstructive than obstructed epicardial coronary vessels. The one year mortality rate of patients with obstructive coronary artery disease is considered at 3.9%, however patients with MVA considered lower at 1% [26].Death rates in patients with chronic stable symptoms ranges with and without obstructive lesions at 0.6% and 2.0% per year respectively [27,28]. However prognosis is much poorer if the symptoms are due to infiltrative processes such as amyloid or myeloma and if left bundle branch block is present there may be development of cardiomyopathy [29].

This chapter will look at current ideas regarding MVA including microvascular circulation abnormalities, endothelial dysfunction, sympathetic over activity, metabolic derangement, abnormal pain perception, effects of oestrogen, role of inflammation and current treatment strategies.

Measures of Microvascular Flow

Direct measures of microvascular flow are not quite as simple or straight forward as diagnostic studies of epicardial coronary arteries. The following is intended as a succinate summary of the most widely used techniques rather than an exhaustive review. We will consider invasive, none invasive imaging and peripheral flow mediation methods of assessing microvascular flow. There are other methods including some experimental techniques that are beyond the scope of this review chapter.

Blood flow to regional myocardial vascular beds can be measured allowing myocardial perfusion and more importantly any deficits between rest and stress to be assessed. Blood flow during rest and stress are compared, in order to obtain the most accurate compensatory effect, maximal coronary dilatation is required. This is achieved by intravenous inotropes and vasodilators. Myocardial blood flow may increase by four fold during stress when compared to rest [30]. This may lead to supply and demand mismatches resulting in myocardial ischemia. This perfusion deficit can be measured directly using specialised guide wires that have sensors at their tip such as Doppler, thermistor or pressure sensors. We can then calculate a ratio of blood flow under stress and rest the so called coronary flow reserve (CFR) [31,32,33,34,207] thereby allowing any myocardial microvascular deficiency to become identified. If present, further assessments are performed with Doppler and or thermo dilution [30]. One of these techniques called coronary flow reserve (CFR) measures the flow response further downstream of the microvascular bed allowing direct assessment of coronary microvascular function during infusion of endothelial dependant and independent vasodilators directly into coronary epicardial arteries [35,36,37,38]. These Invasive strategies allow direct measures of microvascular flow resistance. They are useful indexes of myocardial flow. Therefore if a reduced coronary blood flow is seen in the context of normal coronary arteries by either ultrasound or fractional flow reserve, it can be concluded that this is due to dysfunction in the microcirculation [39]. Development of dual sensor pressure and flow wires has allowed the direct measure of coronary flow reserve.This has allowed more detailed information regarding coronary perfusion physiology [32,40,41]. There is debate whether such invasive and time consuming techniques have a role [19,29]. However, the WISE study found that major adverse cardiac events were more prevalent in those women with a CFR of less than 2.32 [42]. These included nonfatal myocardial infarction, nonfatal stroke, congestive heart failure and death [42].

Invasive measures were taken as gold standard, however, recent advances in non-invasive imaging techniques allow reliable myocardial perfusion and therefore CFR to be calculated[43]. There are a number of non-invasive modalities available for microvascular assessment. We will consider briefly SPECT studies, PET, cardiac CT and MRI modalities.Single photon emission tomography (SPECT) stress myocardial perfusion for people who are to exercise or the use of dipyridamole or adenosine-induced vasodilation in conjunction with SPECT imaging or echocardiography in patient that cant exercise[44,45,46]. These techniques do not permit direct measures of blood flow but rather allow only comparisons of perfusion during resting and stressed states [47].Others such as computed tomography (CT), echo Doppler, quantitative contrast echocardiography, and PET allow tissue perfusion measurements. However, one important issue for all these techniques are that they do not assess the microcirculation independently from epicardial[48,49,50]. Despite the inability for direct measurements, great deal of information can still be made. If we consider 2 vascular beds each consisting of an epicardial coronary artery supplying blood to a vascular bed via coronary microvascular bed. For example if we consider 2 vascular systems each consisting of an epicardial artery supplying a microvascular bed with one of these systems consisted of an epicardial artery with a stenosis, and the other system with an unobstructed epicardial artery. With the flow through both vascular systems being measured, if an intervention is performed on the epicardial artery with a stenosis with subsequent decrease in resistance and an increase in blood flow through the microvascular bed, we can conclude therefore a change in epicardial artery was responsible and not the microcirculation. Similarly, if a decrease in resistance is observed after an intervention in the system without an obstructed epicardial artery then we could extrapolate that this was due to change in the microvasculature rather than the epicardial artery.This same idea therefore can be applied to assess any change in micro vascular bed and assess for possible micro vascular angina [47].

The most accurate non-invasive modality is PET imaging, which has been used for several years for myocardial blood flow assessment. With its improved resolution and ability to perform intrinsic attenuation correction PET scanning allows determination of blood flow and therefore CFR non-invasively [51,52,53]. Patients with abnormal PET scanning CFR calculations (<2.0) with 13N-ammonia are associated with major adverse cardiac effects over the first 3 years when compared to patients with normal CFR calculations [54].

Cardiac CT perfusion imaging uses a bolus of contrast to visualise cardiac vasculature. The method relies on first pass of contrast through the myocardium to obtain most accurate information. The principle is based on calculating contrast concentration and correlating this to the myocardial blood flow. Images taken during rest and stress allow for determination of any perfusion defects but also for myocardial perfusion reserves (MPR). The MPR may be decreased due to significant disease in epicardial vessels and in endothelial dysfunction in epicardial or microvascular circulation [55]. Detailed structural and instantaneous perfusion detail is possible, however, the nephrotoxicity due to iodinated contrast, radiation and the necessity of having to use beta blockers to decrease artefact but decrease accuracy to assess microcirculation [30]. Further research into CT scanning with 320 sections in use of calculating MPR is still underway in the CORE 320 multicentre trial.

Cardiac MR with gadolinium enhancement has been used since 1990s for the assessment of MPR [56,57]. MR assessment of MPR and coronary artery disease is comparable to PET and SPECT imaging respectively [58,59]. A normal MR study is associated with very low cardiac events rate (0.8%) over the next three years [59]. This was further ratified by a study that involved 100 women and found that assessment of LV function with perfusion could identify high risk group that suffered higher rates of MACE events such as recurrent chest pains, myocardial infarctions and even death [60].

Flow mediated dilatation is a peripheral method of measuring coronary microvascular and endothelial function. Kelmsummarised 3 methods in which endothelial function can be measured; the first is a direct measurement of the morphology and mechanical properties of vessel wall. Secondly, measures of endothelial markers and finally focal area of endothelial dependantregulation of vascular tone [61]. Endothelium plays a pivotal role in organ perfusion via blood flow and vascular tone. With increased blood flow vessels dilate in a physiological phenomenon called flow mediated dilatation (FMD) first coined by Schretzenmayer [62]. Celermajer [63] proposed a non-invasive method of assessing FMD in forearm circulation. The method involved applying a cuff around proximal forearm to pressures above systolic blood pressure in effect producing a stenosis in the brachial artery. This leads to a downstream post stenotic dilatation. On release of the pressure cuff a sudden increase of blood flow along the dilated vessels to the vascular bed is seen. Shearing forces are seen upstream which in turn cause dilatation of the brachial artery that can be measure with ultrasound [203]. This response is compared to the response to GTN, the latter being more pronounced. However, in patients with a number of cardiovascular risk factors the effect of GTN is impaired [64]. Therefore, endothelial dysfunction is correlated to an impaired FMD response. High fat meal, postprandial lipaemia [65], mental stress [66], oestrogen and progesterone levels [67], smoking [68], changes in glucose [69], sodium and calcium [70] all acutely influence measures of FMD. Masciet identified a relationship between brachial artery (FMD) and myocardial perfusion. Patients identified with abnormal perfusion defects also had significant lower FMD than those patients with no perfusion deficits. Therefore this seems to suggest a link between endothelial dysfunction and abnormalities of myocardial blood flow in MVA patients [71].

Circulation Abnormalities

Ischemia as the cause of cardiac MVA has on a number of occasions been questioned due to unobstructed coronary arteries on angiography, lack of response with nitrates and negative stress echocardiograms observed in a large number of patients [29,72,73]. Coronary angiography remains the gold standard for assessment of the larger epicardial coronary, with angiography enabling studies of vessels with spatial resolution as small as 0.5mm. However the smaller resistance vessels that are responsible for regulation of the majority of myocardial blood flow are not visualised[30]. If we consider and appreciate that significant coronary artery stenosis disease decreases blood flow distal to the epicardial artery [74]. This is the premise of intervention to open the obstruction and allowing blood flow. However, some authors have observed an association with only mild atherosclerosis and impaired coronary blood flow regulation with in microvascular vessels [75]. What's even more interesting is that not only flow reserve decrease distal within vascular bed of the coronary artery but also decreased flow has been seen in adjacent vascular beds in both experimental animal models and clinical populations [76]. Minimal [77] or intermediate [78] obstructive lesion within epicardial coronary vessels, have been noted to affect global coronary flow reserves. Such lesions also increase the likelihood of development of restenosis after PCI [79].

There have been a number of abnormalities of coronary microvasculature proposed as a possible cause of MVA. One such abnormality that has been put forward is vasospasm at rest or reduced dilatation with exercise that would consequently result in reduced coronary reserves and subsequent ischaemic sounding chest pains and symptoms. This was highlighted in the ACOVA study. This was a prospective study of 304 consecutive patients admitted with angina like chest pains and subsequently had diagnostic coronary angiography, 144 had normal coronary arteries. These patients then went on to have intracoronary acetylcholine and this caused coronary spasm in 77 patients (62%). The coronary vasospasms were epicardial and microvascular in 45% and 55% respectively.Within the epicardial system greater than 75% of diameter lumen reduction was seen in symptomatic patients. Microvascular spasm could not be measured directly and were identified by reproduction of symptoms, ischaemicECG changes in patients with normal epicardial angiography [80]. This study suggests that abnormal vasoreactivity plays a role in pathogenesis of MVA. Acetylcholine has also been noted to cause anterior wall myocardial perfusion defects on scintography due to endothelial dysfunction [81,82].Buchthal et al measured high energy phosphates prior to and after stress testing, they found that 20% of patients had abnormalities that were consistent with myocardial ischaemia[83]. Similarly, Panting et al noted subendocardial hypoperfusion on cardiac MRI with infusion of adenosine [48]. Both of these studies support ischaemia as the pathophysiological mechanism of MVA.

Coronary microvasculature has also been studied and it has been proposed that a decrease of the number of coronary capillaries in patients with MVA. This decreased number of micro vessels is coupled with decreased lumen size of the microvessels. The decreased lumen size was noted to be due to swollen endothelium [84].The significant increase in media thickness was due to fibromuscular thickening seen in endomyocardial biopsies [4] in blood vessels less than 100micrometres in diameter of patient with MVA. This subsequently results in an increase in microvessel wall to lumen diameter ratio [85]. In effect the decreased lumen diameter results in a decrease blood supply to myocardium.Interestingly cutaneous skin biopsies of patients suffering with MVA have shown a significant decrease in skin capillary density [86] just as in the myocardium.

Endothelial Functional Abnormalities

Endothelium mediated vasodilatation dysfunction has been suggested [51,52,79] as a possible cause of MVA. This concept originated from appreciating that stress induced perfusion defects may not be due to myocardial ischaemia or hypoxia as these are only capable of slight reduction in nuclear isotope uptake, however the predominant reason for a stress induced perfusion defect is infactthe differential increase in coronary blood flow from rest to stressed states [88]. Therefore endothelial dysfunction of the coronary circulation may be responsible for myocardial ischaemia during stress testing [81]. Recent studies suggest that endothelial dysfunction is an import cause of both abnormal microcirculation as well as atherosclerosis development [81,90,91].Coronary vascular endothelium has a pivotal role in regulating vasomotor tone by secreting vasoactive substances by either dilating or constricting coronary vasotone. Agents such as prostacyclin, nitric oxide and hyperpolarising relaxing factor collectively known as EDRF maintain myocardial blood flow during periods of increased metabolic demands [91,92,93,94,95]. Atherosclerosis and its associated risk factors impair EDRF activity, and therefore shift the neurohumeral balance towards vasoconstriction [91,92,93]. Multiple factors are involved in auto regulation of coronary blood flow - metabolic, neurohumeral and flow physical changes such as intraluminal pressure or shear stresses [96,97,98]. Therefore changes in endothelial factors may be responsible for myocardial ischaemia in the absence of significant coronary disease [29].The site of microvascular dysfunction is under debate with some studies suggesting that restrictive arterioles [99] having been thought to be the site of endothelial dysfunction, however some authors believe pre-arteriolar dysfunction causing reduced production of endothelium derived relaxing factor [100]. Taking to side the exact vessel responsible, endothelial dysfunction has also been associated with early atherosclerosis, this may contribute to MVA or at least in a subgroup patients [101,102,103].

In order to maintain coronary blood flow despite changes in perfusion pressure the coronary vasculature is able to auto regulate [104,105]. Oxygen and metabolites are important auto regulation factors another is the so called myogenic response which causes constriction in response to increased transmural pressure [106].This mechanism in the face of increasing perfusion pressure prevents excessive flow to coronary vasculature [107,108].Endothelial derived relaxing factor nitric oxide (NO) is made from L-arginine and via stimulating guanylatecyclase within smooth muscle converting GTP-cGMP causes vascular smooth muscle relaxation [109] NO plays a very important role in regulation of coronary vasculature and therefore blood flow both in vivo as well as isolated hearts [110,111,205]. A dramatic example of the potency of NO is commonly seen in septic patients with vascular relaxation being linked with increased release of NO [109]. Interestingly, experimental evidence that NO counteracts the autoregulation by myogenic tone and that the inhibition of NO has been noted to reverse the dysfunction of coronary autoregulation in both rabbit and guinea pig hearts [112,113] again underlining the importance of NO.Reduced bioavailability of nitric oxide as a result of endothelial dysfunction and enhanced expression of endothelin-1, promoted by inflammatory mechanisms, may be implicated in the impairment of systemic endothelial vasoreactivity leading to MVA [114]. NO also plays an important role in the increase in coronary blood flow following coronary arterial occlusion in other words myocardial reactive hyperaemia post myocardial infarcts [115,116]. Massive coronary vasodilatation as mentioned above, due to increase NO production in sepsis disrupts coronary autoregulation and inhibition of L arginine, NO or cGMP pathways results in restoration of coronary autoregulation[117]. Impairment of endothelial mediated vasodilatation was greatly improved with administration of L-arginine, a substrate for NO production, in patients with MVA [118]. Significantly impaired coronary vasodilation was observed by Opherk etal who used dipyridamole, a potent vasodilator in patientswith MVA with some success [119]. Therefore could the syndrome be at least partly explained by this phenomenon [119].

Coronary flow reserve is the ability of quantifying myocardial blood flow, and as mentioned above, is the ratio between maximal stress and rest states with abnormal range 2.0-2.5 [31,32]. CFR can be used for assessment of epicardial arteries but if a decrease in CFR is present despite normal epicardial arteries this decrease is therefore a representation of decrease microvascular flow [30]. CFR is typically decreased in the setting of epicardial stenosis, but in the absence of this, decreased CFR is representative of microvascular dysfunction. Invasive techniques to derive CFR are possible with the use of sensor tipped guidewires to assess rest and stressed blood flow [31,32,33,34]. The WISE trial studied the relationships between major adverse outcomes and baseline CFR by use of intracoronary adenosine in 189 female patients diagnosed with suspected ischaemia. The group demonstrates that invasively assessed decreased CFR (< 2.32) is associated with increased risk of major adverse clinical events, including death, nonfatal myocardial infarction, nonfatal stroke, and heart failure hospitalization. MVA therefore may occur as a result of both endothelium dependent and endothelium-independent dysfunctional flow regulation and be associated with adverse cardiovascular outcomes [42].The study concluded in women with suspected ischaemia and risk factors for atherosclerosis the use of microvascular coronary vasoreactivity to adenosine improved prediction of adverse outcomes than the use of angiographic epicardial disease and atherosclerotic risk factors alone. The significance of microvascular coronary vessels was not only highlighted but the study also concluded that future work should be aimed at microvascular vessel as potential targets for diagnosis and treatment of MVA [42].

Sub study from the WISE study noted that 61 women with normal diagnostic coronary angiography and coronary flow reserve (CFR) <3.0 after adenosine were assigned to either ACE-I (quinalpril was used in this trial) or a placebo group. The CFR was then assessed 16 weeks later.The microvascular function improved in the former group and was associated with reduction in angina.The greatest improvements were noted in patient with the lower baselines at start of the study [120]. Yet another sub group study of WISE showed improvement in CFR with inhibition of phosphodiesterase type 5 (100mg oral sildenafil) The CFR was tested before and 45 minutes after oral sildenafil. The response was noted in women with a CFR < 2.5 however no improvement was seen in women with CFR > 2.5. The group suggested that randomised trials with longer term effects of inhibition were needed [121].

Initially it was felt that this abnormality mainly resulted in reduced vasodilator capacity in response to metabolically active stimuli. Experimental and clinical findings have shown active vasoconstriction of coronary vessels during stress testing in myocardial regions with reduced flow and regional hypoperfusion [122,123,124].The phenomena seen during coronary angiography of slow transit of contrast that is usually seen in one coronary vessel has been observed by some authors in all 3 epicardial vessels has been referred to as "slow flow" [4,5].This phenomenon may also be associated with chest pain and ST segment and has been noted on scintography to cause myocardial perfusion deficit. Interestingly, nitrates did not reverse the perfusion deficit however papaverine an arteriolar dilator appeared to alleviate both symptoms and ST changes [125].This phenomenon coupled with studiesshowing medial hypertrophy of myocardial microvessels appears to support the hypothesis of excessive constriction of restrictive arterioles [5]. These findings were further validated by the use of intracoronary administration of neuropeptide Y a sympathetic co-transmitter. The mechanism by which neuropeptide Y causes arteriolar vasoconstriction remains unknown. The precise pathophysiology is unknown howeveran increased level of endothelin-1, a potent microvascular constrictor that is synthesised by endothelium, has been seen in cardiac MVA [126]. Interestingly the same group also noted an abnormal response of the microvasculature in these patients [127]. Cannon et al also paced patients with MVA and noted decreased ability of these patients to reduce coronary vascular resistance which would suggest inability to vasodilatation. The group also proposed that agents may be present that may affect coronary microvasculature causing constriction or limit vasodilatation [99].

Role of Inflammation

There have been a number of studies correlating inflammatory processes to acute coronary syndromes via plaque inflammation from release of cytokines that may be able to activate endothelium thereby transforming antiaggregant and anticoagulant substrate to aggregate and procoagulant ones [128,129]. They have also been associated with reduced matrix synthesis and increased degradation therefore favouring plaque rupture [128,129]. Increased CRP and tissue endothelial 1 like immune response at localised sites of unstable plaques [130] suggesting vasoreactivity of localised plaque due to inflammation processes

[131]. There has been recent evidence to suggest a correlation between elevated CRP, a marker for both acute phase and chronic inflammation, with vascular abnormalities in patients with MVA [132,133,134,203]. The inflammatory response is thought to contribute to or cause endothelial dysfunction. Inflammation has also been linked with reduced bioavailability and enhanced expression of nitric oxide and endothelin-1, leading to impaired vasoreactivity [134]. Therefore many authors believe that increased endothelins and decreased nitric oxide lead to increased vasoconstriction and decreased vasodilatation respectively. This may be the pathophysiological mechanism for MVA.

Patients with coronary artery disease and high CRP exhibited reduced forearm vasodilator response to acetylcholine than patients with coronary artery disease with normal CRP concentrations [135]. Interestingly normalisation of CRP was associated with vasodilator response, therefore suggesting a correlation between inflammation and microvascular endothelial dysfunction due to inability to vasodilate[135]. The relationship between endothelial dysfunction and CRP is also seen in healthy patients with early atherogenesis, as investigated by Cleland et al who measured basal forearm blood flow in healthy individuals with normal and elevated CRP [136]. Those patients with elevated CRP had decrease forearm blood flow. Furthermore Cosin etal studied 137 patients (33 of who were male) with a mean age 57 years that experienced chest pain but had normal coronary angiography. The patients underwent exercise testing, 24 hour Holter monitors and CRP measurements. The study noted a correlation between elevated CRP in patients with higher frequency, longer duration of symptoms and in patients with ST segment depression on exercise testing or Holter monitoring than those patients with less frequent symptoms and no ECG changes on either Holter monitoring or exercise stress testing [134].Tomai et al [130] studied patients with unstable angina and noted that in patients with increased CRP concentrations they exhibited an attenuation of changes in minimal epicardial coronary artery diameter during the cold pressor testing. This seemed to suggest that increased CRP concentration was associated with enhanced vasoreactivity at the site of the obstructive lesion.

Teragawa studied 46 patients with normal coronary angiograms and divided them into 2 groups based on CRP concentrations. The two groups either had normal or elevated CRP. Baseline coronary artery diameter and coronary blood flow was similar in both sub groups. Challenges of acetylcholine, a marker of endothelial dysfunction, was then infused into the left coronary artery for 2 minutes. They found that coronary blood flow increased in patients with elevated CRP, however this response was not observed in patients with normal CRP [137]. Patients with MVA had higher levels of CRP, increased carotid artery media thickness and increased stiffness of the carotid arteries, therefore a possible link between inflammatory process and vascular abnormalities [138]. Going a step further a recent study by Ong et al investigated brachial artery FMD, high sensitivity CRP (hs-CRP) and obesity. The team found that MVA patients had high BMI, impaired brachial artery FMD and significantly elevated hs-CRP.More interestingly was a correlation between impaired brachial artery FMD, hs CRP and obesity in patients with MVA. In other words low grade inflammation and obesity may in some manner give rise to vascular dysfunction [139] and therefore MVA.

Sympathetic Overactivity
and Metabolic Abnormalities

Shortly after ischaemia was first proposed as the pathophysiological mechanism accounting for MVA, a numberof investigators started to observe abnormal neural regulation as the pathophysiological base of MVA [140,141,142,143,144]. Increased stimulation of adrenergic receptors within the coronary blood vessels by sympathetic nervous system has also been documented [53].Heart rate variability studies demonstrated an increase of sympathetic outflow to myocardium resulting in increased oxygen demand of myocardium as well as constriction of epicardial and microvascular blood vessels thereby reducing coronary flow reserves [145]. Several authors have also proposed thathyperdynamic blood pressure and heart rate in patients are seen in MVA patients [140,141,146].The effects may not be as severe as to cause an ST elevation myocardial infarct, however the effects may be more subtle such as the observation of impaired diastolic dysfunction, impaired relaxation, seen in MVA patients [144,147,148]. However, the authors were unable to conclude if the effect was due to or consequence of cardiac MVA. Moreover, it has been appreciated that both symptoms and diastolic function are note to improve with long term beta blockers [147] suggestive a causative link.Beta blockers reduce circulating fatty acids and in doing so shift the balance to increase carbohydrate metabolism. Therefore it has been suggested that beta blockers improve diastolic function by re-establishing normal myocardial metabolism [149].

Myocardial metabolism in MVA patients has been observed to have reduced carbohydrate utilisation with an increase in lipid fuels [7,142]. This was seen in a study that paced MVA patients that were noted to have a net production of pyruvate due to lactate formation as a result of lipid metabolism, a metabolic process that is promoted by sympathetic drive [140]. This was not seen in normal patients that preferentially metabolised carbohydrates [140].Metabolic response to stress testing assessed by phosphorous-31 nuclear magnetic resonance spectroscopy was first seen in a study by Buchthal who noted that 20% of women with syndrome X had abnormal metabolic response during stress [83]. Buffon et al measured lipid hydroperoxidases and conjugated dienes which are sensitive and independent markers of ischaemia reperfusion oxidative stress. They measure the above markers before and after pacing induced tachycardia and found that in patients with MVA there was a large release of products of lipid peroxidation similar to patients with known ischaemia[150].

In periods of prolonged fasting fatty acid and ketone levels increase by lipolysis to provide substrate for metabolism. During fasting blood sugar and insulin levels are reduced. However, in cardiac MVA patients glucose levels continue to be high as seen by positron imaging of fluorine 18-deoxyglucose that traces trans-membrane glucose transport. This is another pathophysiological mechanism that has been observed to be reversed to normal metabolism by prolong beta blocker use. This abnormal glucose uptake and metabolism is also observed in patients with myocardial ischemia seen in areas of under perfusion during myocardial perfusion tomography. Therefore seems to suggest myocardial ischaemia causing chest pain in syndrome MVA [151] Increased sympathetic tone may also cause increased regional uptake of glucose [150] as well interstitial deposition of gadolinium [148]. DTPA has also been seen to accumulate on MRI scanning, within myocardial regions that have high glucose uptake and again can also be seen to accumulate in area of myocardial ischaemia. This is further highlighted by the fact that increased DTPA uptake is reduced by prolonged use of beta blockers [148]. Insulin resistance may also be caused by adrenergic receptors; this phenomenon may be reversed by use of beta blocker (propranolol was the beta blocker used in this study) that leads to normal glucose uptake [152]. Insulin resistance has been linked with reduction in endothelial derived relaxing factor [153,154,155] therefore abnormal vasoconstriction in MVA; leading to ischaemia, therefore excessive sympathetic activity may cause or at least contribute to insulin resistance [156,157].

The role of sympathetic over activity has been questioned by some authors such as Galassi who showed that prazocin had no improved effects on patients exercise duration or number of episodes of ST depression on Holter monitor [143]. Similarly Rosen et al also found that doxazocin an alpha block had no effect on coronary vasodilator reserve [158] and the observation that cold pressor stimulation that should induce alpha 1 mediated vaso-constriction [159] had no difference in effect between normal patients compared to cardiac MVA patients [160]. Could parasympathetic impairment rather than sympathetic over activity have a role? Gulli et al tested heart rate variability in time and frequency domains together by looking at spectral analysis finger arterial pressure with bedside autonomic tests. They found that a vagal (parasympathetic) impairment seen in MVA patients that were not present in normal patients [161]. However further studies did not show significant difference between vagal activity in MVA and normal patients [161,162,163].

Abnormal Pain Perception

It is widely believed that MVA patients seem to have heightened myocardial sensitivity [164,165]. Ballon inflation or electrical pacing within the right atrium, normally a painless procedure has been noted to be a painful stimuli in cardiac MVA patients [165]. Shapiro et al investigated pain perception in patients with MVA by injecting saline into atria. In patients with MVA found this to be a painful stimulus [164] however in asymptomatic patient with non-obstructed epicardial vessels had no associated pain. 29 patients with MVA underwent quantitative measurements of myocardial perfusion with 15O labelled water with infusion of dipyridamole and compared the perfusion images during stress to the images during rest. No significant differences were seen when compared to a matched population of control group. Of interest was the fact that dipyridamole infusion caused pain in the majority of MVA patients as well as ST changes in a third of these patients. The research group therefore cast doubt of ischaemia as the cause of pain in syndrome x patients, however they stressed the importance of sympathetic activation as a possible cause for the pain [168].

Abnormal pain reception due to altered endogenous opioid system in MVA patients has been proposed[167]. Lanza et al found that a significant proportion of MVA patients had regional and even global abnormalities or both in cardiac meta-iodobenzylguanidine (MIBG) scintigraphy, suggesting an abnormal efferent function of cardiac sympathetic nerve endings [168]. Rosen et al performed brain PET scanning in patients with MVA during episodes of pain and found that greater extent of cortical activation particularly in right anterior insular than in patients with episodes of angina that had coronary artery disease [169].In attempt to summarise the complex role of pain perception in MVA patients Sylven et al suggested that there existed a complex interaction between the dysregulatedcardiac nervous system, propitiating sympathetic drive and a central neurogenic component [170].

It has become accepted that abnormalities in visceral pain perception are seen in MVA patients; however no clear evidence exists as to how far up the afferent nervous system the abnormalities extend. The dysregulation may extend right up to the cortical level of the central nervous system and or involve the endogenous opioid system [167]. This is highlighted by the fact that targeting of central nervous system pain perception may prove to be more successful than traditional anti-anginal therapy at least in some patients[171,172].

Oestrogen

The syndrome, as mentioned above, is more prevalent in women than in men, and furthermore the vast majority of women with MVA are peri- or postmenopausal [173]. This has led to the possibility of a link to oestrogen. Postmenopausal women with MVA have abnormal endothelial function, which is improved by the administration of oestrogen. Thus oestrogen deficiency has been postulated to have a pathogenic role in MVA [174,175].Low oestrogen levels have been associated with impaired function of the endogenous opioid system that controls pain perception. Therefore low oestrogen levels may be responsible for the reduction or suppression of the production and or release of endorphins and encephalins. This is turn leading to increased pain perception and may contribute to the symptoms of cardiac MVA [176,177].

Patient Management

Despite the syndrome not having such a benign prognosis as first thought many patients with MVA have good long term prognosis [9,29], although many patients have poor quality of life due to symptoms [173].Life style measures should be encouraged. Exercise and rehabilitation has been shown to increases pain thresholds, encourage endothelial function and therefore delays onset of pain [178]. The exact mechanism is not understood.It has been long been appreciated that chronic smoking has a greater effect on endothelial vasoreativity than hypertension or hypercholesterolemia [91] and therefore smoking cessation should be a priority.

The current established treatment has been targeted towards atherosclerosis-associated comorbidities, such as hypertension and hyperlipidaemia [179].However there have been no large scale studies validating current treatment lines. There is however some evidence that aggressive treatment of hypertension is associated with decreased cardiac events due to endothelial function recovery [180].Improved endothelial function has also been demonstrated with angiotensin-converting enzyme (ACE-i) inhibitors [181,182] and benefit as also been observed with the use of statins, independent on effect of lipid profile [183,184,185,186]. Both of these have been associated with decrease or delay onset of exertional induced chest pain [187.188].Many other medications that are used in angina are also been beneficial in view of symptoms in patient with MVA such as beta blockers [189,190] nitrates [191] and calcium channel blockers [192]. Tricyclic antidepressants [193], oestrogen replacement therapy [114] L-arginine [194,195,196] and aminophylline being associated with improvements in symptoms [197] these stress multifactorial and complex nature of the syndrome. More recently, imipramine has been used to increase patient pain perception [193,198,199]. Oestrogen has not been recommended for long term therapy for chronic conditions including MVA [200].Psychological therapies have also been of great benefit [201], with particular focus on Cognitive behavioural therapy [202]. Finally, Spinal cord stimulation has also been tied in refractory patients. This technique acts via dorsal pain gate control area and has been observed to improve angina symptoms in MVA patients [202,204].

Conclusion

First being described over 40 years ago as cardiac syndrome xthen a decade latter as MVA, this phenomenon of patients with cardiac sounding chest pain, demonstrated ischaemia on stress testing but without obstructive lesions seen within epicardial coronary arteries on diagnostic angiography.Despite being a remarkably common syndrome with a greater prevalence in females, remains still an under recognised syndrome that has more recently proved to have an associated mortality and morbidity. Initially thought due to myocardial ischaemia, the exact pathophysiology still eludes us today. This perhaps suggest that the syndrome is likely multifactorial in origin. Mirocovascular circulation abnormalities, endothelial dysfunction, sympathetic over activity, abnormal pain perception, effects of oestrogen, and inflammation have all been suggested as possible etiological mechanisms. The possible varied origins of this syndrome is reflected in current treatment practices that relate largely to symptoms, not only with the use of statins, ACE- inhibitors, nitrates, calcium channel blockers, beta blockers, tricyclic antidepressants, L-arginine, spinal cord stimulation and even cognitive behavioural therapy. Great emphasis is also being placed on rehabilitation with symptoms decreasing with greater exercise. Smoking cessation also needs to be a high priority.Much progress has been made over the last 40 years with the condition becoming more recognised and therefore diagnosed. Despite lack of current national or international guidelines patients are being treated according to best current evidence. We are currently in a very exciting time with a number of researchers eluding the complex pathophysiology of the syndrome and this will lead to development of best medical management of such patients.

References

[1]   Likoff W, Segal BL, Kasparian H: Paradox of normal selective coronary arteriograms in patients considered to have unmistakable coronary heart disease. *N Engl J Med* 1967, 276:1063–1066.

[2]   Kemp HG, Jr.: Left ventricular function in patients with the anginal syndrome and normal coronary arteriograms. *Am J Cardiol* 1973, 32:375–376.

[3]   Cannon RO, Watson RM, Rosing DR, Epstein SE: Angina caused by reduced vasodilator reserve of the small coronary arteries. *J Am CollCardiol* 1983, 1:1359–1373.

[4] Mosseri M, Yarom R, Gotsman MS, Hasin Y. Histologic evidence for small-vessel coronary artery disease in patients with angina pectoris and patent large coronary arteries. *Circulation* 1986; 74: 964-72.

[5] Przybojewski JZ, Becker PH. Angina pectoris and acute myocardial infarction due to 'slow-flow phenomenon' in nonatherosclerotic coronary arteries: a case report.

[6] Maseri A. The changing face of angina pectoris. Practical implications. *Lancet* 1983; 1: 746-9.

[7] Cannon RO, Camici PG, Epstein SE. Pathophysiological dilemma of syndrome X. *Circulation* 1992;85:883–92

[8] Davis KB, Chaitman B, Ryan T, et al. Comparison of 15-year survival for men and women after initial medical or surgical treatment for coronary artery disease: a CASS registry study. *J Am CollCardiol* 1995;25:1000–9.

[9] Kaski JC. Pathophysiology and management of patients with chest pain and normal coronary arteriograms (cardiac syndrome X). *Circulation* 2004;109:568–572.

[10] Bugiardini R, BaireyMerz CN. Angina with 'normal' coronary arteries: a changing philosophy. *JAMA* 2005;293:477–484.

[11] Lanza GA. Cardiac syndrome X: a critical overview and future perspectives. *Heart* 2007;93:159–166.

[12] Diver DJ, Bier JD, Ferreira PE etal: Clinical and CurrCardiol Rep (2011) 13:151–158 155 arteriographic characterization of patients with unstable angina without critical coronary arterial narrowing (from the TIMI-IIIA Trial). *Am J Cardiol*1994, 74:531–537.

[13] Phibbs B, Fleming T, Ewy GA, etal: Frequency of normal coronary arteriograms in three academic medical centers and one community hospital. *Am J Cardiol*1988, 62:472–474.

[14] Kemp HG, Kronmal RA, VlietstraRE,etal: Seven year survival of patients with normal or near normal coronary arteriograms: a CASS registry study. *J Am CollCardiol* 1986, 7:479–483.

[15] Sullivan AK et al (1994) Chest pain in women: clinical, investigative, and prognostic features. *BMJ* 308(6933):883–886.

[16] Gielen S, Schuler G, Hambrecht R. Exercise training in coronary artery disease and coronary vasomotion. Circulation 2001;103:E1–E6.

[17] Tuzcu EM, Kapadia SR, Tutar E, Ziada KM, Hobbs RE, McCarthy PM et al. High prevalence of coronary atherosclerosis in asymptomatic teenager and young adults: evidence from intravascular ultrasound. *Circulation* 2001;103:2705–2710.

[18] Arslanian-Engoren C et al (2006) Symptoms of men and women presenting with acute coronary syndromes. *Am J Cardiol* 98(9):1177–1181.

[19] Canto JG et al (2007) Symptom presentation of women with acute coronary syndromes: myth vs reality. *Arch Intern Med* 167(22):2405–2413.

[20] DeVon HA, Zerwic JJ (2002) Symptoms of acute coronary syndromes: are there gender differences? A review of the literature. *Heart Lung* 31(4):235–245.

[21] Cunningham MA et al (1989) The effect of gender on the probability of myocardial infarction among emergency department patients with acute chest pain: a report from the Multicenter Chest Pain Study Group. *J Gen Intern Med* 4(5):392–398.

[22] Kudenchuk PJ et al (1996) Comparison of presentation, treatment, and outcome of acute myocardial infarction in men versus women (the Myocardial Infarction Triage and Intervention Registry). *Am J Cardiol* 78(1):9–14.

[23] Milner KA et al (2002) Typical symptoms are predictive of acute coronary syndromes in women. *Am Heart J* 143(2):283–288.

[24] Milner KA et al (1999) Gender differences in symptom presentation associated with coronary heart disease. *Am J Cardiol* 84(4):396–399.

[25] Shaw LJ et al (2006) The economic burden of angina in women with suspected ischemic heart disease: results from the NationalInstitutes of Health—National Heart, Lung, and Blood Institute—sponsored Women's Ischemia Syndrome Evaluation. *Circulation* 114(9):894–904.

[26] Bugiardini R, Manfrini O, De Ferrari GM. Unanswered questions for management of acute coronary syndrome: risk stratification of patients with minimal disease or normal findings on coronary angiography. *Arch Intern Med* 2006;166:1391–1395.

[27] Johnson BD, Shaw LJ, Pepine CJ, Reis SE, Kelsey SF, Sopko G et al. Persistent chest pain predicts cardiovascular events in women without obstructive coronary artery disease: results from the NIH-NHLBI-sponsored Women's Ischaemia Syndrome Evaluation (WISE) study. *Eur Heart J* 2006;27:1408–1415.

[28] Daly C, Clemens F, Lopez Sendon JL, Tavazzi L, Boersma E, Danchin N et al. Gender differences in the management and clinical outcome of stable angina. *Circulation* 2006;113:490–498).

[29] Kaski JC, Rosano GM, Collins P, Nihoyannopoulos P, Maseri A, Poole-Wilson PA. Cardiac syndrome X: clinical characteristics and left ventricular function. Long-term follow-up study. *J Am CollCardiol.* 1995;25:807–814.

[30] Vesely MR,Dilsizian V; Microvascular Angina: Assessment of Coronary Blood Flow, Flow Reserve, and Metabolism, *CurrCardiol Rep* (2011) 13:151–158

[31] Kern MJ, de Bruyne B, Pijls NH: From research to clinical practice: current role of intracoronary physiologically based decision making in the cardiac catheterization laboratory. *J Am CollCardiol*1997, 30:613–620

[32] Kern MJ: Coronary physiology revisited : practical insights from the cardiac catheterization laboratory. Circulation 2000, 101:1344–1351.Ziadi M, Beanlands R: The clinical utility of assessing myocardial blood flow using positron emission tomography. *J NuclCardiol*2010, 17:571–581

[33] Doucette JW, Corl PD, Payne HM, Flynn AE, Goto M, Nassi M, Segal J: Validation of a Doppler guide wire for intravascular measurement of coronary artery flow velocity. *Circulation* 1992,85:1899–1911

[34] Melikian N, Kearney MT, Thomas MR, De Bruyne B, Shah AM, MacCarthy PA: A simple thermodilution technique to assess coronary endothelium-dependent microvascular function in humans: validation and comparison with coronary flow reserve.*Eur Heart J* 2007, 28:2188–2194

[35] Bugiardini R, Manfrini O, Pizzi C, Fontana F, Morgagni G. Endothelial function predicts future development of coronary artery disease: a study of women with chest pain and normal coronary angiograms. *Circulation*2004;109:2518–2523.

[36] Suwaidi JA, Hamasaki S, Higano ST; etal Long-term follow-up of patients with mild coronary artery disease and endothelial dysfunction. *Circulation* 2000;101:948–954.

[37] Schachinger V, Britten MB, Zeiher AM. Prognostic impact of coronary vasodilator dysfunction on adverse long-term outcome of coronary heart disease. *Circulation* 2000;101:1899–1906.

[38] Halcox JP, Schenke WH, Zalos G, Mincemoyer R, Prasad A, Waclawiw MA et al. Prognostic value of coronary vascular endothelial dysfunction. *Circulation* 2002;106:653–658.

[39] Fearon WF, Nakamura M, Lee DP, Rezaee M, et al. Simultaneous assessment of fractional and coronary flow reserves in cardiac transplant recipients: Physiologic Investigation for Transplant Arteriopathy (PITA Study). *Circulation* 2003;108:1605–1610.

[40] Baumgart D, Haude M, Liu F, Ge J, Goerge G, Erbel R. Current concepts of coronary flow reserve for clinical decision making during cardiac catheterization. *Am Heart J* 1998;136:136–149.

[41] Siebes M, Verhoeff BJ, Meuwissen M, de Winter RJ, Spaan JA, Piek JJ. Single-wire pressure and flow velocity measurement to quantify coronary stenosis hemodynamics and effects of percutaneous interventions. *Circulation* 2004;109:756–762.

[42] Pepine C, Anderson R, SharafB,etal : Coronary microvascular reactivity to adenosine predicts adverse outcome in women evaluated for suspected ischemia results from the National Heart, Lung and Blood Institute WISE (Women's Ischemia Syndrome Evaluation) study. *J Am CollCardiol* 2010, 55:2825–2832.

[43] Schelbert H: Anatomy and physiology of coronary blood flow. *J NuclCardiol* 2010, 17:545–554.

[44] Hachamovitch R, Berman DS, Kiat H, Cohen I, Friedman JD, Shaw LJ. Value of stress myocardial perfusion single photon emission computed tomography in patients with normal resting electrocardiograms: an evaluation of incremental prognostic value and cost-effectiveness. *Circulation* 2002;105:823–829.

[45] Bartel T, Yang Y, Muller S, Wenzel RR, Baumgart D, Philipp T et al. Noninvasive assessment of microvascular function in arterial hypertension by transthoracic Doppler harmonic echocardiography. *J Am CollCardiol*2002;39:2012–2018.

[46] Poelaert JI, Schupfer G. Hemodynamic monitoring utilizing transesophageal echocardiography: the relationships among pressure, flow, and function. *Chest* 2005;127:379–390.

[47] Pries AR, Helmut HabazettlH,AmbrosioG, etalA review of methods for assessment of coronary microvascular disease in both clinical and experimental settings. *Cardiovascular Research* (2008) 80, 165–174.

[48] Panting JR, Gatehouse PD, Yang G-Z, et al. Abnormal subendocardial perfusion in cardiac syndrome X detected by cardiovascular magnetic resonance imaging. *N Engl J Med.* 2002;346:1948–1953.

[49] Doyle M, Fuisz A, Kortright E, Biederman RW, Walsh EG, Martin ET et al. The impact of myocardial flow reserve on the detection of coronary artery disease by perfusion imaging methods: an NHLBI WISE study. *J Cardiovasc Magn Reson* 2003; 5:475–485.

[50] Wagner B, Anton M, Nekolla SG, Reder S, Henke J, Seidl S et al. Noninvasive characterization of myocardial molecular interventions by integrated positron emission tomography and computed tomography. *J Am CollCardiol*2006;48:2107–2115.

[51] Quyyumi AA, Cannon RO III, Panza JA, Diodati JG, Epstein SE. Endothelial dysfunction in patients with chest pain and normal coronary arteries. *Circulation* 1992; 86: 1864-71.

[52] Egashira K, Inou T, Hirooka Y, Yamada A, Urabe Y, Takeshita A. Evidence of impaired endothelium-dependent coronary vasodilatation in patients with angina pectoris and normal coronary angiograms. *N Engl J Med* 1993; 3281 1659-64

[53] Montorsi P, Fabbiocchi F, Loaldi A el al. Coronary adrenergic hyperactivity in patients with syndrome X and abnormal electrocardiogram at rest. *Am J Cardiol* 1991; 68: 1698-703.

[54] Herzog BA, Husmann L, Valenta I, Gaemperli O et al: Long-term prognostic value of 13 N-ammonia myocardial perfusion positron emission tomography added value of coronary flow reserve. *J Am CollCardiol* 2009, 54:150–156.

[55] Schuleri K, George R, Lardo A: Assessment of coronary blood flow with computed tomography and magnetic resonance imaging. *J NuclCardiol*2010, 17:582–590. This manuscript reviews the current progress, future outlook as well as strengths and limitations of noninvasive quantitative myocardial perfusion imaging by CT and MRI methodologies.

[56] Wilke N, Jerosch-Herold M, Wang Y;Myocardial perfusion reserve: assessment with multisection, quantitative, first-pass MR imaging. *Radiology* 1997, 204:373–384.

[57] Atkinson DJ, Burstein D, Edelman RR: First-pass cardiac perfusion: evaluation with ultrafast MR imaging. *Radiology* 1990, 174:757–762.

[58] Fritz-Hansen T, Hove JD, Kofoed KF, Kelbaek H, Larsson HB: Quantification of MRI measured myocardial perfusion reserve in healthy humans: a comparison with positron emission tomography. *J MagnReson Imaging* 2008, 27:818–824.

[59] Schwitter J, Wacker CM, van Rossum AC,et al.: MR-IMPACT: comparison of perfusioncardiac magnetic resonance with single-photon emission computed tomography for the detection of coronary artery disease in a multicentre, multivendor, randomized trial. *Eur Heart J*2008, 29:480–489.

[60] Doyle M, Weinberg N, Pohost G, et al.: Prognostic value of global MR myocardial perfusion imaging in women with suspected myocardial ischemia and no obstructive coronary disease: results from the NHLBI-sponsored WISE (Women's Ischemia Syndrome Evaluation) study. *JACC Cardiovasc Imaging* 2010, 3:1030–1036.

[61] Kelm, M; Flow-mediated dilatation in human circulation: diagnostic and therapeutic aspects; Am J Physiol Heart CircPhysiol 282:H1-H5, 2002.

[62] Schretzenmayer A (1933) überKreislaufregulatorischeVorgängean den grossen Arterienbei der Muskelarbeit. *Pflügers Arch* 232:S743–S748.

[63] Celermajer DS, Sorensen KE, Gooch VM, etal. Non-invasive detection of endothelial dysfunction in children and adults at risk of atherosclerosis. *Lancet* 340: 1111–1115, 1992.

[64] Adams MR, Robinson J, Celermajer DS; etal Smooth muscle dysfunction occurs independently of impaired endothelium-dependent dilation in adults at risk of atherosclerosis. *J Am CollCardiol*32: 123–127, 1998.

[65] Evans M, Anderson RA, Graham J; etalCiprofibrate therapy improves endothelial function and reduces postprandial lipemia and oxidative stress in type 2 diabetes mellitus. *Circulation* 101: 1773–1779, 2000.

[66] Ghiadoni L, Donald AE, Cropley M etal; Mental stress induced transient endothelial dysfunction in humans. *Circulation* 102: 2473–2478, 2000.

[67] Sorensen KE, Dorup I, Hermann AP etal; Combined hormone replacement therapy does not protect women against the age-related decline in endothelium-dependent vasomotor function. *Circulation* 97: 1234–1238, 1998.

[68] Lekakis J, Papamichael C, Vemmos C, Effect of acute cigarette smoking on endothelium-dependent brachial artery dilatation in healthy individuals. *Am J Cardiol* 79: 529–531, 1997.

[69] Kawano H, Motoyama T, Hirashima O, Hyperglycemia rapidly suppresses flow-mediated endothelium-dependent vasodilation of brachial artery. *J Am CollCardiol* 34: 146–154, 1999.

[70] Bevan JA. Flow regulation of vascular tone. Its sensitivity to changes in sodium and calcium. *Hypertension* 22: 273–281, 1993)

[71] Masci PG, Laclaustra M, Lara JG, Kaski JC. Brachial artery flow-mediated dilation and myocardial perfusion in patients with cardiac syndrome X. *Am J Cardiol.* 2005;95: 1478–1480.

[72] Kaski JC. Cardiac syndrome X and microvascular angina. In: *Chest Pain With Normal Coronary Angiograms: Pathogenesis, Diagnosis and Management.* Edited by Kaski . London: Kluwer Academy Publishers; 1999. pp. 1–12.

[73] Nihoyannopoulos P, Kaski JC, Crake T, Maseri A. Absence of myocardial dysfunction during stress in patients with syndrome X. *J AmCollCardiol.* 1991;18:1463–1470.

[74] Zeiher AM, Drexler H, Wollschlager H, Just H. Modulation of coronaryvasomotor tone in humans. Progressive endothelial dysfunction with different early stages of coronary atherosclerosis. *Circulation* 1991;83:391–401.

[75] Schachinger V, Britten MB, Elsner M, Walter DH, Scharrer I, Zeiher AM. A positive family history of premature coronary artery disease is associated with impaired endothelium-dependent coronary blood flow regulation. *Circulation* 1999;100:1502–1508.

[76] Sambuceti G, Marzullo P, Giorgetti A, Neglia D, Marzilli M, Salvadori P et al. Global alteration in perfusion response to increasing oxygen consumption in patients with single-vessel coronary artery disease. *Circulation* 1994;90:1696–1705.

[77] Britten MB, Zeiher AM, Schachinger V. Microvascular dysfunction in angiographically normal or mildly diseased coronary arteries predicts adverse cardiovascular long-term outcome. *Coron Artery Dis* 2004;15: 259–264.

[78] Chamuleau SA, Tio RA, de Cock CC, de Muinck ED, Pijls NH, van Eck-Smit BL et al. Prognostic value of coronary blood flow velocity and myocardial perfusion in intermediate coronary narrowings and multivessel disease. *J Am CollCardiol* 2002;39:852–858.

[79] Haude M, Baumgart D, Verna E, Piek JJ, Vrints C, Probst P et al. Intracoronary Doppler- and quantitative coronary angiography-derived predictors of major adverse cardiac events after stent implantation. *Circulation* 2001;103:1212–1217.

[80] Ong P, Athanasiadis A, Borgulya G etalHigh Prevalence of a Pathological Response to Acetylcholine Testing in Patients With Stable Angina Pectoris and Unobstructed Coronary Arteries The ACOVA Study (Abnormal COronaryVAsomotion in patients with stable angina and unobstructed coronary arteries) *J Am CollCardiol.* 2012 Feb 14;59(7):655-62.

[81] Hasdai D, Gibbons RJ, Holmes DR, et al. Coronary endothelialdysfunction in humans is associated with myocardial perfusion defects. *Circulation* 1997;96:3390–5).

[82] Zeiher AM, Krause T, Schächinger V, et al. Impaired endothelium-dependent vasodilation of coronary resistance vessels is associated with exercise-induced myocardial ischemia. *Circulation* 1995;91:2345–52

[83] Buchthal SD, den Hollander JA, Merz CN, et al. Abnormal myocardial phosphorus-31 nuclear magnetic resonance spectroscopy in women with chest pain but normal coronary angiograms. *N Engl J Med.* 2000;342:829–835

[84] Mosseri M, Schaper J, Admon D, et al. Coronary capillaries in patients with congestive cardiomyopathy or angina pectoris with patent main coronary arteries – ultrastructural morphometry of endomyocardial biopsy samples. *Circulation.*1991;84:203–210

[85] Bund SJ, Tweddel A, Hutton I, HeagertyAM. Small artery structural alterations of patients with microvascular angina. *Clin Sci.* 1996;91:739–743

[86] Antonios TF, Kaski JC, Hasan KM, Brown SJ, Singer DR. Rarefaction of skin capillaries in patients with anginal chest pain and normal coronary arteriograms. *Eur Heart J.* 2001;22: 1144–1148.

[87] Motz W, Vogt M, Rabenay O, Scheler S, Luckhoff A, Straver BE. Evidence of endothelial dysfunction in coronary resistance vessels in patients with angina pectoris and normal coronary angiograms. *Am J Cardiol* 1991; 68: 996-1003.

[88] Verani SV. Stress echocardiography versus nuclear imaging. In: Zaret BL, Beller GA, eds. *Nuclear cardiology – state of the art and future directions.* New York: CV Mosby, 1999:368–78

[89] Zeiher AM, Drexler H, Saurbier B, et al. Endothelium-mediated coronary blood flow modulation in humans: effects of age, atherosclerosis, hypercholesterolemia, and hypertension. *J Clin Invest* 1993;92:652–62.

[90] Toborek M, Kaiser S. (1999) Endothelial cell functions. Relationship to atherogenesis. *Basic Res Cardiol* 94:295–314.

[91] Drexler H. Endothelial dysfunction: clinical implications. *ProgCardiovasc Dis* 1997;4:287–324.

[92] Moncada S, Gryglewski RJ, Bunting S, et al. An enzyme isolated from arteries transform prostaglandin endoperoxidase to an unstable substance that inhibit platelet aggregation. *Nature* 1976;263:663–5.

[93] Furchgott RF, Zawadzki JV. The obligatory role of endothelial cells in the relaxation of arterial smooth muscle by acetylcholine. *Nature* 1980;288:373–6

[94] Vane R, Anggard EE, Botting RM. Regulatory functions of the vascular endothelium. *N Engl J Med* 1990;323:27–36

[95] Zeiher AM, Drexler H, Wollschläger H, et al. Coronary vasomotion in response to sympathetic stimulation in humans: importance of functional integrity of the endothelium. *J Am CollCardiol* 1989;14:1181–90

[96] DeFily DV, Chilian WM. Coronary microcirculation: autoregulation and metabolic control. *Basic Res Cardiol* 1995;90:112–18.

[97] Muller JM, Davis MJ, Chilian WM. Integrated regulation of pressure and flow in the coronary microcirculation. *Cardiovasc Res* 1996;32:668–78

[98] Kuo L, Davis MJ, Chilian WM. Myogenic activity in isolated subepicardial and subendocardial coronary arteries. *Am J Physiol*1988;255:H1558–62

[99]   Cannon RO, Bonow RO, Bacharach SL et al. Left ventricular dysfunction in patients with angina pectoris, normal epicardial coronary arteries and abnormal vasodilator reserve. *Circulation* 1985; 71: 218-26

[100] Maseri A, Crea F, Kaski JC, Crake T. Mechanisms of angina pectoris in syndrome X. *J Am CollCardiol*1991; 17: 499-506

[101] Thorne S, Mullen MJ, Clarkson P, Donald AE, Deanfield JE. Early endothelial dysfunction in adults at risk from atherosclerosis: differentresponses to L-arginine. *J Am CollCardiol*1998;32:110–116.

[102] Lerman A, Holmes DR Jr, Bell MR, Garratt KN, Nishimura RA, Burnett JC Jr. Endothelin in coronary endothelial dysfunction and early atherosclerosis in humans. *Circulation* 1995;92:2426–2431.

[103] Zeiher AM, Drexler H, Wollschlager H, Just H. Endothelial dysfunction of the coronary microvasculature is associated with coronary blood flow regulation in patients with early atherosclerosis. *Circulation* 1991;84: 1984–1992.

[104] Dole WP. Autoregulation of the coronary circulation.*ProgCardiovasc Dis* 1987;29: 293–323.

[105] Feigl EO. Coronary physiology. Physiol Rev 1983;63:1–205.

[106] Johnson PC. The myogenic response. In: Bohr DF, Somlyo AP, Sparks HV Jr, editors. Handbook of physiology, sect 2: The cardiovascular system, vol II. Vascular smooth muscle, ch 15. Bethesda, MD: *The American Physiological Society,* 1981;409–442.

[107] Aukland K, Nicolaysen G. Interstitial fluid volume: Local regulatory mechanisms. *Physiol Rev* 1981;61:556–643.

[108] Davis MJ. Microvascular control of capillary pressure during increases in local arterial and venous pressure. *Am J Physiol*1988;254:H772–H784.

[109] Moncada S, Palmer RM, Higgs EA. Nitric oxide: physiology, pathophysiology, and pharmacology. *Pharmacol Rev* 1991;43:109–142.

[110] Amezcua JL, Palmer RM, de Souza BM, Moncada S. Nitric oxide synthesized from L-arginine regulates vascular tone in the coronary circulation of the rabbit. *Br J Pharmacol* 1989;97:1119–1124.

[111] Chu A, Chambers DE, Lin CC, et al. Effects of inhibition of nitric oxide formation on basal vasomotion and endothelium-dependent responses of the coronary arteries in awake dogs. *J Clin Invest* 1991;87:1143–1149.

[112] Pohl U, Lamontagne D, Bassenge E, Busse R. Attenuation of coronary autoregulation in the isolated rabbit heart by endothelium derived nitric oxide. *Cardiovasc Res* 1994;28:414–419.

[113] Ueeda M, Silvia SK, Olsson RA. Nitric oxide modulates coronary autoregulation in the guinea pig. *Circ Res* 1992;70:1296–1303.

[114] Rosano GM, Peters NS, Lefroy D,: 17-beta-Estradiol therapy lessens angina in postmenopausal women with syndrome X. *J Am CollCardiol* 1996, 28:1500–1505.

[115] Kostic MM, Schrader J. Role of nitric oxide in reactive hyperemia of the guinea pig heart. *Circ Res* 1992;70:208–212.

[116] Yamabe H, Okumura K, Ishizaka H, Tsuchiya T, Yasue H. Role of endothelium derived nitric oxide in myocardial reactive hyperemia. *Am J Physiol* 1992;263:H8–H14.

[117] Avontuur J, Bruining H, Can Ince C; Nitric oxide causes dysfunction of coronary autoregulation in endotoxemic rats. *Cardiovascular Research* 35 _1997. 368–376

[118] Egashira K, Hirooka Y, Kuga T, Mohri M, Takeshita A. Effects of L-arginine supplementation on endothelium-dependent coronary vasodilatation in patients with angina pectoris and normal coronary arteriograms. *Circulation*. 1996;94:130–134).

[119] Opherk D, Zebe H, Wiehe E, et al. Reduced coronary dilatory capacity and ultra-structural changes of the myocardium in patients with angina pectoris but normal coronary arteriograms. *Circulation*. 1981;63:817–825.

[120] Pauly DF, Johnson BD, Anderson RD etalIn women with symptoms of cardiac ischemia, nonobstructive coronary arteries, and microvascular dysfunction, angiotensin-converting enzyme inhibition is associated with improved microvascular function: A double-blind randomized study from the National Heart, Lung and Blood Institute Women's Ischemia Syndrome Evaluation (WISE) *Am Heart J*. 2011 Oct;162(4):678-84.

[121] Denardo SJ, Wen X, Handberg EMEffect of phosphodiesterase type 5 inhibition on microvascular coronary dysfunction in women: a Women's Ischemia Syndrome Evaluation (WISE) ancillary study *ClinCardiol*. 2011 Aug;34(8):483-7. doi: 10.1002/clc.20935.

[122] Sambuceti G, Marzili M, Maraccini P, et al. Coronary vasoconstriction during myocardial ischemia induced by rises in metabolic demand in patients with coronary artery disease. *Circulation* 1997;95:2652–9.

[123] Guyton RA, McClenathan JH, Newman GE, et al. Evolution of regional ischemia distal to a proximal coronary stenosis: self-propagation of ischemia. *Am J Physiol* 1985;248:H403–11.

[124] Gorman MW, Sparks HV. Progressive coronary vasoconstriction during relative ischemia in canine myocardium. *Circ Res* 1982;51:411–20.

[125] Chierchia S, Margonato A, Fragasso G, Gerosa S. Microvascular spasm can cause ischaemia in patients with normal coronary arteries (Abstr). *Circulation* 1990; 82: III-248.

[126] Kaski JC, Elliott PM, Salomone O, et al. Concentration of circulating plasma endothelin in patients with angina and normal coronary angiograms. *Br Heart J*. 1995;74:620–624.

[127] Cox ID, Botker HE, Bagger JP, Sonne HS, Kristensen BO, Kaski JC. Elevated endo-thelin concentrations are associated with reduced coronary vasomotor responses in patients with chest pain and normal coronary arteriograms. *J Am CollCardiol*. 1999;34:455–460.

[128] Libby P, Ridker PM, Maseri A. Inflammation and atherosclerosis. *Circulation*2002;105:1135–43.

[129] Crea F , Biasucci LM, Buffon A, et al. Role of inflammation in the pathogenesis of unstable coronary artery disease. *Am J Cardiol*1997;80 (5A) :10E–16E.

[130] TomaiF ,Crea F, Gaspardone A, et al. Unstable angina and elevated c-reactive protein levels predict enhanced vasoreactivity of the culprit lesion. *Circulation* 2001;104:1471–6).

[131] BogatyP , Hackett D, Davies G, et al. Vasoreactivity of the culprit lesion in unstable angina. *Circulation*1994;90:5–11.

[132] Desideri G , Gaspardone A, Gentile M, et al. Endothelial activation in patients with cardiac syndrome X. *Circulation* 2000;102:2359–64

[133] TousoulisD , Davies GJ, Asimakopoulos G, et al. Vascular cell adhesion molecule-1 and intercellular adhesion molecule-1 serum level in patients with chest pain and normal coronary arteries (syndrome X). *ClinCardiol*2001;24:301–4.

[134] Cosin Sales J, Pizzi C, Brown S, Kaski JC. C-reactive protein, clinical presentation and ischemic activity in patients with chest pain and normal coronary angiograms. *J Am CollCardiol.* 2003;41:1468–1474.

[135] FichtlschererS , Rosenberger G, Walter DH, et al. Elevated C-reactive protein levels and impaired endothelial vasoreactivity in patients with coronary artery disease. *Circulation*2000;102:1000–6.

[136] Cleland SJ, Sattar N, Petrie JR, et al. Endothelial dysfunction as a possible link between C-reactive protein levels and cardiovascular disease. *ClinSci*2000;98:531–5.

[137] Teragawa H, Fukuda Y, Matsuda K. Relation between C reactive protein concentrations and coronary microvascular endothelial function. *Heart.* 2004;90:750–754.

[138] Arroyo-Espliguero R, Mollichelli N, Avanzas P, et al. Chronic inflammation and increased arterial stiffness in patients with cardiac syndrome X. *Eur Heart J.* 2003;24:2006–2011

[139] Ong P, Sivanathan R, Borgulya G etal Obesity, Inflammation and Brachial Artery Flow-Mediated Dilatation: Therapeutic Targets in Patients with Microvascular Angina (Cardiac Syndrome X) Cardiovasc Drugs Ther. 2012 Mar 6 epub ahead of print.

[140] Arbogast R, Bourassa MG. Myocardial function during atrial pacing autonomic control of the cardiovascular system in syndrome X. Am in patients with angina pectoris and normal coronary arteriograms. *J Cardiol* 1994;73:1174–1179.

[141] Romeo F, Gaspardone A, Ciavolella M, Gioffre P, Reale A. Verapamil versus acebutalol for syndrome X. *Am J Cardiol* 1988;62:312–313.

[142] Camici PG. Marraccini P, Lorenzoni R el al. Coronary hemodynamics and myocardial metabolism in patients with syndrome X: Response to pacing stress. *J Am CollCardiol* 1991; 17: 1461-70.

[143] Galassi AR, Kaski J-C, Pupita G, Vejar M, Crea F, Maseri A. Lack of evidence for alpha-adrenergic receptor-mediated mechanisms in the genesis of ischemia in syndrome X. *Am J Cardiol* 1989;64:264– 269.

[144] Spinelli L, Ferro G, Genovese A, Cinquegrana G, Spadafora M, Condorelli M. Exercise-induced impairment of diastolic time in patients with X syndrome. *Am Heart J* 1990;119:829–833.

[145] Rosen SD. Guzzetti S, Mezzetti S, Lombardi F, Camici PG, Malliani A. Altered pattern of circadian neural control of heart rate period in syndrome X*Eur Heart J* 1993: 14 (AbstrSuppl): 429.

[146] Camici PG, Marraccini P, Lorenzoni R et al. Coronary hemodynamics and myocardial metabolism in patients with syndrome X: response to pacing stress. *J Am CollCardiol* 1991;17:1461–1470.

[147] Fragasso G, Pizzetti G, Carlino M et al. Chronic betablockade reverses diastolic dysfunction in patients with syndrome X (Abstr). *J Am CollCardiol 1993*; 21: 253A.

[148] Rossetti E, Fragasso G, Vanzulli A et al. Magnetic resonance imaging in patients with angina and normal coronary angiograms. *J Am CollCardiol* 1994; (Spec issue): 445A.

[149] Chierchia SL,Fragasso GAngina with normal coronary arteries: diagnosis, patho-physiology and treatment. *European Heart Journal* (1996) 17 {Supplement G), 14-19).

[150] Buffon A, Rigattieri S, Santini SA, et al. Myocardial ischemiareperfusion damage after pacing-induced tachycardia in patients with cardiac syndrome X. *Am J Physiol Heart Circ Physiol.* 2000;279.

[151] Fragasso G, Chierchia SL, Conversano A, Lucignani G, Landoni C, Fazio F. Myocardial anaeorobic glycolysis in patients with angina and normal coronary arteries. *Circulation* 1990; 82: 111-249.

[152] Deibert DC, De Fronzo RA. Epinephrine-induced insulin essential hypertension. N Engl J Med 1990; 323: 22-6. resistance in man. *J Clin Invest* 1980; 65: 717-21.

[153] De Tejada IS, Goldstein I, Azadzio K, Krane RJ. Cohen RA. Impaired neurogenic and endothelium-mediated relaxation of penile smooth muscle from diabetic men with impotence. *N Engl J Med* 1989; 320: 1025-30

[154] Panza JA, Quyyumi AA, Brush JE, Epstein SE. Abnormal endothelium-dependent vascular relaxation in patients with essential hypertension. *N Engl J Med* 1990; 323: 22-6.

[155] Smooth cell proliferation in man by insulin Pfeide B, Ditschuneit H Effect of insulin on growth of cultured human arterial smooth muscle cells. *Diabetologia*1981, 20: 155-8.

[156] Dean JD. Jones CJH, Hutchison SJ. Peters JR, Henderson AH. Hyperinsulinaemia and microvascular angina ('syndrome X). *Lancet* 1991; 337: 456-7.

[157] Julius S. Sympathetic hyperactivity and coronary risk in [41] Panza JA, Quyyumi AA, Brush JE, Epstein SE. Abnormal hypertension. *Hypertension* 1993; 21: 886-93.

[158] Rosen SD, Boyd HL, Lorenzoni R, Kaski J-C, Foale RA, Camici PG. Effect of a - adrenoceptor blockade on coronary vasodilator reserve in cardiac syndrome X. *J CardiovascPharmacol*1999;34:554–560.

[159] Nabel EG, Ganz P, Gordon JB, Alexander AW, Selwyn AP. Dilatation of normal and constriction of atherosclerotic coronary arteries caused by the cold pressor stimulation. *Circulation* 1988;77:43–52.

[160] Meeder JG, Blanksma PK, van der Wall EE et al. Coronary vasomotion in patients with syndrome X: evaluation with positron emission tomography and parametric myocardial perfusion imaging. *Eur J Nucl Med* 1997;24:530–537.

[161] Gulli G, Pancera P, Menegatti G, Vassanelli C, Cevese A. Evidence of parasympathetic impairment in some patients with cardiac syndrome X. *Cardiovasc Res* 2001;52:208–216.

[162] Meeder JG, Blanksma PK, Crijns HJGM et al. Mechanisms of angina pectoris in syndrome X assessed by myocardial perfusion dynamics and heart rate variability. *Eur Heart J* 1995;16:1571–1577.

[163] Frobert O, Molgaard H, Botker HE, Bagger JP. Autonomic balance in patients with angina and a normal coronary angiogram. *Eur Heart J* 1995;16:1356–1360.

[164] Shapiro LM, Crake T, Poole-Wilson PA. Is altered cardiac sensation responsible for chest pain in patients with normalcoronary arteries? Clinical observations during cardiac catheterization.*BMJ.* 1988;296:170–171.

[165] Cannon RO, Quyyumi AA, Schenke WH et al. Abnormal cardiac sensitivity in patients with chest pain and normal coronary arteries. *J Am CollCardiol*1990;16:1359–1366.

[166] Rosen SD, Uren NG, Kaski JC, Tousoulis D, Da vies GJ, Camici PG. Coronary vasodilator reserve, pain perception, and sex in patients with syndrome X. *Circulation* 1994; 90: 50-60.

[167] Fedele F, Agati L, Pugliese M, et al. Role of the central endogenous opiate system in patients with CSX. *Am Heart J.* 1998;136:1003–1009.

[168] Lanza GA, Giordano A, Pristipino C, et al. Abnormal cardiac adrenergic nerve function in patients with syndrome X detected by metaiodobenzylguanidine myocardial scintigraphy. *Circulation.* 1997;96:821–826.

[169] Rosen SD, Paulesu E, Frackowiak RSJ, Camici PG. Regional brain activation compared in angina pectoris and syndrome X. *Circulation* 1995;92:I-651.

[170] Eriksson B, Svedenhag J, Martinsson A, Sylve´n C. Effect of epinephrine infusion on chest pain in syndrome X in the absence of signs of myocardial ischemia. *Am J Cardiol* 1995;75:241–245.

[171] Cannon RO. The sensitive heart. A syndrome of abnormal cardiac pain perception. *J Am Med Assoc* 1995;273:883–887.

[172] Potts SG, Lewin R, Fox KA, Johnstone EC. Group psychological treatment for chest pain with normal coronary arteries. *Q J Med* 1999;92:81–86.

[173] Kaski J etal. Cardiac syndrome X: pathogenesis and management. *Heart Metab.* 2008; 40:30–35.

[174] Kaski JC. Cardiac syndrome X in women: the role of oestrogen deficiency. *Heart.* 2006;92 (suppl 3):5–9.

[175] RoqueM, Heras M, Roig E, et al. Short-term effects of transdermal estrogen replacement therapy on coronary vascular reactivity in postmenopausal women with angina pectoris and normal results on coronary angiograms. *J Am Coll Cardiol.*1998;31:139–143.

[176] Kennedy SE, Zubieta JK. Neuroreceptor imaging of stress and mood disorders. *CNS Spectr.* 2004;9:292–301.

[177] Zubieta JK, Smith YR, Bueller JA, et al. Regional mu opioid receptor regulation of sensory and affective dimensions of pain. *Science.* 2001;293:311–315.

[178] Eriksson BE, Tyni-Lenne R, Svedenhag J, et al. Physical training in syndrome X: physical training counteracts deconditioning and pain in syndrome X. *J Am CollCardiol.* 2000;36:1619– 1625.

[179] Braunwald E, Antman EM, Beasley JW et al.: ACC/AHA 2002 guideline update for the management of patients with unstable angina and non-STsegment elevation myocardial infarction—summary article: a report of the American College of Cardiology/American Heart Association task force on practice guidelines (Committee on the Management of Patients With Unstable Angina). *J Am CollCardiol* 2002, 40:1366–1374.

[180] ModenaMG, Bonetti L, Coppi F, Bursi F, Rossi R: Prognostic role of reversible endothelial dysfunction in hypertensive postmenopausal women. *J Am CollCardiol* 2002, 40:505–510.

[181] Kaski JC, Rosano G, Gavrielides S, Chen L: Effects of angiotensin-converting enzyme inhibition on exercise-induced angina and ST segment depression in patients with microvascular angina. *J Am CollCardiol* 1994, 23:652–657.

[182] Chen JW, Hsu NW, Wu TC, Lin SJ, Chang MS: Long-term angiotensin-converting enzyme inhibition reduces plasma asymmetric dimethylarginine and improves endothelial nitric oxide bioavailability and coronary microvascular function in patients with syndrome X. *Am J Cardiol*2002, 90:974–982.

[183] Simaitis A, Laucevicius A: Effect of high doses of atorvastatin on the endothelial function of the coronary arteries. *Medicina* (Kaunas) 2003, 39:21–29.

[184] Kayikcioglu M, Payzin S, Yavuzgil O, Kultursay H, Can LH, Soydan I: Benefits of statin treatment in cardiac syndrome-X1. *Eur Heart J* 2003, 24:1999–2005.

[185] Houghton JL, Pearson TA, Reed RG: Cholesterol lowering with pravastatin improves resistance artery endothelial function: report of six subjects with normal coronary arteriograms. *Chest* 2000, 118:756–760.

[186] Caliskan M, Erdogan D, GulluH : Effects of atorvastatin on coronary flow reserve in patients with slow coronary flow. *ClinCardiol*2007, 30:475–479.

[187] Kaski JC, Valenzuela Garcia LF. Therapeutic options for the management of patients with cardiac syndrome X. *Eur Heart J.* 2001;22:283–293.

[188] Braunwald E, Antman E, Beasley J, et al. ACC/AHA guidelines for the management of patients with unstable angina and non- ST segment elevation myocardial infarction – executive summary and recommendations. A report of the American College of Cardiology/American Heart Association task force on practice guidelines (Committee on the Management of Patients With Unstable Angina). *Circulation.* 2000; 102:1193–1209.

[189] Lanza GA, Stazi F, Colonna G, Pedrotti P, Manzoli A, Crea F, Maseri A: Circadian variation of ischemic threshold in syndrome X. *Am J Cardiol* 1995, 75:683–686.

[190] Ugiardini R, Borghi A, Biagetti L: Comparison of verapamil versus propranolol therapy in syndrome X. *Am J Cardiol*1989, 63:286–290.

[191] Lanza GA, Manzoli A, Bia E, Crea F, Maseri A: Acute effects of nitrates on exercise testing in patients with syndrome X. Clinical and pathophysiological implications. *Circulation* 1994, 90:2695–2700.

[192] Cannon RO, Watson RM, Rosing DR, Epstein SE: Efficacy of calcium channel blocker therapy for angina pectoris resulting from small-vessel coronary artery disease and abnormal vasodilator reserve. *Am J Cardiol* 1985, 56:242–246.

[193] Cannon RO, Quyyumi AA, Mincemoyer R, etal : Imipramine in patients with chest pain despite normal coronary angiograms. *N Engl J Med* 1994, 330:1411–1417.

[194] Lerman A, Burnett JC, Higano ST,: Long-term L-arginine supplementation improves small-vessel coronary endothelial function in humans. *Circulation* 1998, 97:2123–2128.

[195] Fujita H, Yamabe H, Yokoyama M: Effect of L-arginine administration on myocardial thallium-201 perfusion during exercise in patients with angina pectoris and normal coronary angiograms. *J NuclCardiol* 2000, 7:97–102.

[196] Dilsizian V: The role of myocardial perfusion imaging in vascular endothelial dysfunction. *J NuclCardiol* 2000, 7:180– 184.

[197] Elliott PM, Krzyzowska-Dickinson K,etal: Effect of oral aminophylline in patients with angina and normal coronary arteriograms (cardiac syndrome X). *Heart* 1997, 77:523–526.

[198] Aminophylline adenosine receptor antagonist Elliott PM, Krzyzowska-Dickinson K, Calvino R, Hann C, Kaski JC. Effect of oral aminophylline in patients with angina and normal coronary arteriograms (cardiac syndrome X). *Heart.* 1997;77:523–526.

[199] Yoshio H, Shimizu M, Kita Y, et al. Effects of short-term aminophylline administration on cardiac functional reserve in patients with syndrome X. *J Am CollCardiol.* 1995;25: 1547–1551.

[200] Paoletti R, Wenger NK. Review of the international position on women's health and menopause: a comprehensive approach. *Circulation.* 2003;107:1336–1339.

[201] Potts SG, Bass C. Chest pain with normal coronary arteries: psychological aspects. In: Kaski JC, ed. *Chest Pain With Normal Coronary Arteries: Pathogenesis, Diagnosis and Management*. Boston, MA: Kluwer Academic Publishers; 1999. pp. 13–32.

[202] Mayou RA, Bryant BM, Sanders D, Bass C, Klimes I, Forfar C. A controlled trial of cognitive behavioural therapy for noncardiac chest pain. *Psychol Med*. 1997;27:1021–1031.

[203] Tondi P, Santoliquido A, Di Giorgio A et al Endothelial dysfunction as assessed by flow-mediated dilation in patients with cardiac syndrome X: role of inflammation. *Eur Rev Med Pharmacol Sci*. 2011 Sep;15(9):1074-7.

[204] Lanza GA, Sestito A, Sgueglia GA, et al. Effect of spinal cord stimulation on spontaneous and stress-induced angina and "ischemia-like" ST-segment depression in patients with cardiac syndrome X. *Eur Heart J*. 2005;26:983–989.

[205] Feigl EO. Coronary physiology. *Physiol Rev* 1983;63:1–205.

[206] Kern MJ, Lerman A, Bech JW, De BB, Eeckhout E, Fearon WF et al. Physiological assessment of coronary artery disease in the cardiac catheterization laboratory: a scientific statement from the American Heart Association Committee on Diagnostic and Interventional Cardiac Catheterization, Council on Clinical Cardiology. *Circulation* 2006;114:1321–1341.

In: Current Issues in the Management of Stable Ischemic Heart ...   ISBN: 978-1-62417-203-8
Editor: Mukesh Singh   © 2013 Nova Science Publishers, Inc.

Chapter VIII

Contemporary Management of Refractory Angina Pectoris

Mukesh Singh, Tejaskumar Shah, Maunank Patel, Zahid Siddiqui and Sandeep Khosla*

Chicago Medical School, Rosalind Franklin University of Medicine and Science,
North Chicago, Illinois, US

Abstract

Improvements in the treatment of acute coronary syndromes along with increasing prevalence of cardiovascular risk factors including diabetes and obesity have led to increasing population of patients with stable ischemic heart disease. A significant number of these continue to have severe angina despite medical management and revascularization procedures performed. Recently, European society of cardiology joint study group has published strict criteria to define refractory angina. This article reviews the recent advances in clinical evaluation and management strategies for patients with refractory angina.

Background

An estimated 6.4 million patients in the United States suffer from symptomatic coronary artery disease (CAD), and about 400,000 new cases develop each year [1]. With improving treatment modalities for acute coronary syndromes and, thus, outcomes, more patients survive the acute event and their disease state changes into a chronic phase. Also with increasing survival of patients with primary coronary events after revascularization procedures, the number of patients presenting with coronary artery disease unsuitable to further

---

* Address for correspondence: Mukesh Singh, MD. Department of Cardiology. Mt Sinai Hospital Medical Center, 1500 S California Avenue, Chicago, Il-60608, U.S. Fax: 7732576276; Email: drmukeshsingh@yahoo.com.

revascularization techniques and symptoms refractory to medical therapy also continues to rise [2]. In addition, the increasing incidence of cardiovascular risk factors such as diabetes mellitus and obesity combined with the increasing number of revascularization procedures and decreased cardiac mortality rate have transformed the demographic of patients with ischemic heart disease into a steadily increasing population of patients with chronic, and occasionally refractory, angina pectoris. Despite the increasing success of conventional medical treatment and the continued development and improvement of mechanical revascularization approaches, a significant number of patients (5–10%) continue to have severe angina [3].

What Is Refractory Angina?

The European Society of Cardiology (ESC) Joint Study Group on the Treatment of Refractory Angina [4] defines refractory angina as "a chronic condition (>3 months) characterized by the presence of angina caused by coronary insufficiency in the presence of CAD, which is not amenable to a combination of medical therapy, angioplasty, or coronary bypass surgery" in patients with objective evidence of ischemia. Reasons for being a poor candidate for further revascularization include diffuse atherosclerosis, unsuitable anatomy, multiple prior procedures – percutaneous coronary intervention (PCI) or coronary artery bypass graft (CABG) – lack of conduits, absence of reasonable targets for bypass surgery, significant co morbidities such as severe left ventricular (LV) dysfunction, chronic kidney disease, carotid artery disease, and advanced age. It is noteworthy to mention, that sometimes a patient who is labeled as "not suitable candidate for revascularization" might undergo revascularization by another operator. Therefore, the potential for revascularization should be evaluated by other operators before putting the patient in the refractory angina category [5]. Patients with refractory angina have either marked limitation of ordinary physical activity or are unable to perform any ordinary physical activity without discomfort (Canadian Cardiovascular Society [CCS] functional class III or IV). Before diagnosing a patient with RAP, repeated attempts at 'optimizing' medical treatment and lifestyle modification (initiation of an exercise program and discontinuation of tobacco) should be made. Additionally, all secondary causes of angina, such as anemia and uncontrolled hypertension, should be excluded [6].Thus, in order to define refractory angina, several criteria should be met: presence of angina for more than 3 months, objective evidence of reversible ischemia, and exhaustion of ordinary means for treating angina including medical therapy, angioplasty, and coronary bypass surgery [4].

Epidemiology

The epidemiology of refractory angina pectoris is not clearly defined, but estimation depict that >100,000 patients may be diagnosed each year in United States [7]. The European Society of Cardiology estimates as many as 15% of patients with angina have a diagnosis of refractory angina [8].

There is limited data regarding the natural history of refractory angina. Henry et al recently reported an overall mortality of 11.7% (6.2% cardiovascular) at a mean follow-up of 5.4 years in 1,098 patients with refractory ischemia followed at the Minneapolis Heart Institute [9]. This indicates that the major challenge for these patients is not high mortality but persistent angina and poor quality of life.

Management Options

Myocardial ischemia occurs due to a mismatch between myocardial oxygen supply and demand. The main determinants of myocardial oxygen consumption are heart rate, myocardial contractility, wall stress, and fatty acid uptake [10,11]. First step in the management of patients with RA is to determine and treat secondary causes of angina such as hypertension, hyperthyroidism, anemia, hypoxia, continued tobacco use in addition to optimizing the medical management. However, despite an increasing success in multidisciplinary approach of medical therapies and revascularization approaches, refractory angina pectoris continues to pose a significant health problem. As the mortality from CAD decreases, and the population ages, an increasing number of patients will be diagnosed with RA.

Despite many recent therapeutic advances, patients with RA are not adequately treated and suffer from poorly controlled symptoms. This results in end-stage CAD characterized by a severe myocardial insufficiency usually leading to impaired left ventricular function. These patients continue to experience residual anginal symptoms and require frequent hospitalization. A multi-disciplinary approach to the care of these patients has potential to improve angina relief and the quality of life. In addition to traditional therapies, a number of newer treatment modalities have been developed during the last few decades that may be helpful in the management of patients with RA.

Goals of Therapy in RA

The goals for treatment of angina pectoris include symptom relief and risk reduction of future adverse cardiovascular events such as myocardial infarction and death. Similar to other patients with atherosclerotic CAD, the major determinants of reduced survival in patients with RA include older age, male gender, reduced left ventricular ejection fraction, severity of coronary disease, previous MI, and diabetes mellitus [12].

Therefore, medical treatments for this patient population should be divided in two groups with separate goals, therapies that stabilize atherosclerosis and prevent disease progression, recurrent coronary events, preserve left ventricular function, and improve overall survival and therapies that reduce the anginal threshold by decreasing oxygen demand or by improving hemodynamics to increase myocardial oxygen supply. Table 1 lists the goal of therapy and modalities used in RA.

Therapies for Prevention of Recurrent Coronary Events and Improve Survival

Patients with refractory angina should have their cardiac risk factors treated aggressively with secondary prevention measures, and should be on an optimal regimen of antiplatelet and antianginal medications. There is considerable evidence that lifestyle changes and pharmacologic treatment may reduce the progression of atherosclerosis and stabilize plaque in patients with chronic stable angina. Therefore, risk factor modification should be the central component of management [13]. Suggested lifestyle changes include cessation of smoking, exercise and weight reduction, in addition to treatment of hypertension and glycemic control in patients with diabetes. The suboptimal management of cardiovascular risk factors in secondary prevention contributes to high rates of recurrent coronary events in patients with a history of myocardial infarction. Current evidence from multiple clinical trials indicates that aspirin, beta blockers, statins, and ACE inhibitors should be used in nearly all patients with CAD who do not have specific contraindications. This is especially true for patients with a history of myocardial infarction. It has been estimated that up to 85% of recurrent events in patients with coronary disease could be prevented or delayed with the use of these medications [14,15]. It is likely that outcomes could be improved by adding lifestyle modifications such as exercise and dietary changes to the medication regimens [secondary prevention].

Table 1. Goals of therapy and modalities to achieve goals in RA

Goal of Therapy	Therapeutic strategies
Symptom control	A) Traditional agents: Beta blockers, calcium channel blockers, short and long acting nitrates. B) Novel agents: Ranolazine, Nicorandil, Ivabradine, Trimetazidine, Perhexiline, Allopurinol, L-arginine, Fasudil.
Stabilization of Atherosclerosis and prevention of recurrent events	C) Cardiovascular risk factor reduction: healthy lifestyle changes including dietary modification, smoking cessation, exercises, weight loss, control of hypertension and dyslipidemia. D) Drug therapy: Antiplatelet agents, beta blocker, ACE inhibitor, HMG CoA reductase inhibitor (Statins).

Traditional Pharmacological Therapies

Most conventional antianginal agents act by altering cardiovascular hemodynamics, such as a reduction in systemic vascular resistance or coronary vasodilatation or negative inotropism, resulting in improved balance in myocardial oxygen supply and demand. Three major classes of anti-ischemia drugs are currently used in the medical management of angina pectoris: b-blockers, nitrates (short- and long-acting), and calcium channel antagonists (table 1). All three have been shown to prolong the duration of exercise before the onset of angina and ST segment depression as well as to decrease the frequency of angina.

Table 2. Novel anti-anginal agents

Agent	Pharmacological properties	Dose and Side effects	FDA approval for Angina
Ranolazine	• Prevention of calcium overload and the subsequent increase in diastolic tension due to inhibition of late inward sodium channel. • Glycometabolic and antiarrhythmic effects • Hepatic clearance with t1/2 of 2 hours.	• 500 mg BID to 1g BID • Constipation, dizzy, nausea, asthenia, QT interval prolongation, hepatic dysfunction	Yes.
Ivabradine	• Heart rate-lowering agent via I(f) ion channel blockade in SA node • Hepatic clearance with t1/2 of 2 hours.	• 2.5 mg BID to 7.5 mg BID. • Visual disturbance, bradycardia, headache, abdominal discomfort	No.
Nicorandil	• Nitrate-like vasodilation • K ATP channel activation • Inhibition of fatty acid oxidation • Hepatic clearance with t1/2 of 45 minutes.	• 10 mg BID to 30 mg BID; • may use 5 mg BID in patients prone to headache • Headache, GI distress	No.
Allopurinol	• Improves endothelium-dependent vasodilation • reduces xanthine oxidase derived reactive oxidative stress • inhibition of lipid peroxidation , heat shock factor expression, and calcium sensitizing	• Dose for angina not established. • Nausea, diarrhea, hypersensitivity reaction, rash	No
Trimetazidine	• Metabolic modulator increasing myocardial glucose utilization and inhibiting oxidation of fats via 3-ketoacyl coenzyme A thiolase (3-KAT) inhibition • Renal clearance with t1/2 of 6 hours.	• 20 mg 3 times/day with meals • GI intolerance	No
Perhexiline	• Inhibition of fatty acid oxidation	• Start with 100 mg/day and may adjust at 2-4 week intervals; maximum dose: 300-400 mg/day. • Hepatotoxicity, Peripheral neuropathy	No
L-arginine	• Endothelium-dependent vasodilator as a substrate • for nitric oxide (NO) synthase and increased nitric oxide • Hepatic clearance with t1/2 of 1.5-2 hours.	• Dose for angina not established. • Hypotension, hyperkalemia.	No
Fasudil	Rho kinase inhibitor thus modulating vascular smooth muscle contractile response	Investigational agent	No
Molsidomine	nitric oxide donating vasodilator	Investigational agent	No
Testosteroneand Estrogen	Improves endothelial function	Not recommended at present due to concern for adverse effects.	No

Novel Pharmacological Agents

Various novel approaches that have been investigated in order to improve the balance in myocardial oxygen demand and supply include metabolic modulation by inhibiting fatty acid metabolism, ionic channel modulation, reducing reactive oxygen species generation, intracellular signaling modulation and nitric oxide generation. Major novel antianginal agents are mentioned in table 3 and are described below.

Table 3. Non-pharmacological therapies for RA (see text for EECP)

Therapy	Comments
TMR	Invasive percutaneous procedure making 20 to 40 transmural channels using a high-energy carbon dioxide laser with brief manual compression of the epicardial surface to allow for closure of the epicardial opening sites. It stimulates angiogenesis and may destroy nerve fibers to the heart, making patients numb to their chest pain Class IIa indication for RA as per ACC/AHA. Clinical efficacy with 80% response rate in short term but long term follow up not known. Used mainly in conjunction with CABG.
TENS	TENS involves applying a low voltage electrical current via pads placed on the skin in the area of pain. It stimulates large diameter afferent fibers and inhibits input from small diameter fibers in the substantia gelatinosa of the spinal cord. An increased endorphin concentration in blood and cerebrospinal fluid, have also been proposed Advantage: passive, non-invasive, non-addictive modality with no potentially harmful side effect
SCS	SCS blocks pain by stimulating the dorsal columns, which inhibits transmission through the pain-conducting spinothalamic tract. Possible benefits include the ease of use and portability of the device that allows patients to resume activities at home or at work. class IIb indication for treatment of refractory angina as per ACC/AHA guidelines Epidural hematoma and infection, occurring in about 1% of patients. SCS may interfere with pacemakers and implantable defibrillators by possible false inhibition of the pacemaker function, but this risk may be lowered by programming both devices in bipolar mode, and setting the stimulator frequency to 20 Hz.
ESMR	Ultrasound guided shock wave therapy to ischemic areas identified by SPECT. Shockwaves, created by a special generator, are focused using a shockwave applicator device. This induces localized stress on cell membranes, and causes non-enzymatic nitric oxide synthesis from L-arginine and hydrogen peroxide. It also up-regulates VEGF in ischemic myocardium in vivo that causes angiogenesis. The treatment is guided by standard echocardiography equipment. The shockwaves are delivered in synchronization with the patient's R-wave to avoid arrhythmias

Metabolic modulators are agents that exert their effect by increasing the energy available to cardiac cells and improving the metabolic use of cardiac substrates [16]. Under normal conditions in absence of ischemia, the heart uses fatty acids as primary source of energy, since fatty acids produce more ATP than glucose oxidation, but this occurs at the expense of higher oxygen requirement [11,17]. During ischemia, this preferential source of energy utilization is shifted to glucose oxidation – which is more oxygen-efficient and, potentially, may balance the mismatch between oxygen requirement and demand [11,17]. The agents included in this class include ranolazine, Trimetazidine, Nicorandil and Perhexiline.

Ranolazine (approved recently by the US Food and Drug Administration) is a unique anti-ischemic drug that does not significantly affect hemodynamic parameters [18]. It is a piperazine derivative that inhibits the late sodium channels, thereby protecting ischemic myocardial cells by lowering total inward sodium flux and subsequent intracellular calcium overload [19,20]. Combination Assessment of Ranolazine in Stable Angina (CARISA) trial [21] demonstrated that Ranolazine therapy significantly improved exercise duration, time to angina attacks, and electrocardiographic changes indicative of ischemia versus placebo (p<0.01). Ranolazine also significantly reduced the mean weekly anginal attacks and nitroglycerin consumption (p<0.02). This trial showed that ranolazine provided additional antianginal and anti-ischemic efficacy in patients with chronic angina who were symptomatic despite use of other commonly prescribed agents without affecting hemodynamic parameters. Similar results were observed in Monotherapy Assessment of Ranolazine in Stable Angina (MARISA) trial [19] that investigated three doses of sustained-release ranolazine twice daily for 1 week at 500, 1,000, or 1,500 mg. Compared to placebo, all three doses of ranolazine produced a longer time to 1 mm ST-segment depression, increased exercise duration, and lengthened time between anginal attacks.

Trimetazidine is a pure metabolic agent that inhibits free fatty acid beta-oxidation and induces the myocardium to shift from free fatty acids to predominantly glucose utilization in order to increase adenosine triphosphate (ATP) generation per unit oxygen consumption. Trimetazidine in Angina Combination Therapy (TACT) study [22] showed improvement in exercise duration (418 ± 14 to 507 ± 18 seconds vs. 435 ± 15 to 459 ± 16 seconds in the placebo group, p<0.05), time to 1 mm ST depression (389 ± 15 to 480 ± 19 seconds in the treatment group vs. 412 ± 15 to 429 ± 17 seconds in the placebo group, p<0.05), time to onset of anginal pain, mean number of angina attacks per week, and mean consumption of short-acting nitrates per week in favor of trimetazidine [21]. In a Cochrane meta-analysis of 23 studies including 1378 patients, trimetazidine was associated with a significant reduction in weekly angina episodes and improved exercise time to 1 mm ST segment depression compared to placebo [23]. Authors concluded that Trimetazidine is effective in the treatment of stable angina compared with placebo, alone or combined with conventional anti-angina agents [23].

Perhexiline inhibits carnitine palmitoyltransferase-1 (CPT-1) and CPT-2 that are involved in transferring the long free fatty acids across the mitochondrial membrane [24]. Its use is limited by hepatotoxicity and peripheral neuropathy [24,25]. This drug is not currently approved in Europe or the US.

Nicorandil is the only clinically available potassium channel opener with antianginal effects, and with comparable efficacy and tolerability to existing antianginal therapy [26]. Nicorandil is a nicotinamide ester that confers benefits through a dual action: opening the mitochondrial potassium ATP channels leading to preconditioning of the myocardium and a nitrate-like effect [26]. This makes nicorandil a unique antianginal compound that reduces both pre-load and after-load and improves coronary blood flow. Several small randomized trials of patients with stable angina have shown that nicorandil prolongs the time to onset of ST depression and exercise duration during stress testing and improves myocardial perfusion at rest and with exercise [27-30]. Impact Of Nicorandil in Angina (IONA) trial [31] showed that the primary endpoint, a composite of coronary heart disease death, nonfatal MI, or unplanned hospital admission for cardiac chest pain, in patients treated with nicorandil was reduced by 17% (hazard ratio, HR = 0.83, 95% CI, $0.72–0.97; p = 0.014$). Furthermore, the rate of acute coronary syndrome (ACS) was significantly lowered by 21% in the nicorandil treated group (HR: 0.79, 95% CI: 0.64–0.98, p = 0.028) as well as a 14% reduction in all cardiovascular events (HR: 0.86, 95% CI: 0.75–0.98; p= 0.027) [31].

Ivabradine is a selective and specific inhibitor of the I_f ion channel, which is responsible for the primary sino-atrial node pacemaker current [32]. It has the advantage of decreasing heart rate and myocardial oxygen demand without negative inotropic effects. Ivabradine appears to be a safe antianginal agent as a monotherapy or in combination with conventional antianginal medications for the treatment of patients with refractory angina. The benefit and safety of Ivabradine has been demonstrated in combination with other antianginal medications such as beta blockers, nitrates, or calcium-channel blockers [33,34].

Fasudil is an investigational agent that inhibits an intracellular signaling molecule, rho kinase, that is involved in the vascular smooth muscle contractile response. In patients with stable angina, fasudil treatment was demonstrated to significantly increase time to 1 mm ST segment depression, but compared to placebo did not cause any decrease in the time to angina, frequency of angina, or glyceryl trinitrate use [3].

Molsidomine is a nitric oxide donating vasodilator that was shown to reduce the incidence of angina attacks, use of sublingual nitrates, and increased exercise capacity compared to placebo in patients with stable angina. Higher doses provided better protection from angina, but caused hypotension [3].

L-arginine

Both testosterone and estrogen have been shown to improve coronary blood flow in humans. Testosterone acts by endothelium independent mechanisms and may involve the ion channels on vascular smooth muscle cells [35,36], while estrogen improve endothelial function [37,38]. However, concerns exist regarding long-term therapy and side effects both with testosterone (prostate and hematologic effects) and estrogen (initial increase in cardiac events caused by estrogen therapy for females with coronary artery disease) [39]. Therefore these are not the recommended therapies.

Non-Pharmacological Therapies

Although effective in many cases, antianginal medications are insufficient or have side effects in a significant number of patients with severe CAD. For these "no option" patients with RA, the investigation of novel non-pharmacologicaltherapies offers hope for improved quality of life by relieving angina symptoms. Some of the main approaches studied include enhanced external counterpulsation (EECP), transmyocardial laser revascularization (TMR), percutaneous transmyocardial laser revascularization (PTMLR), neuromodulation by transcutaneous electrical nerve stimulation(TENS), spinal cord stimulation (SCS), or stellate ganglion blockade, extracorporeal shockwave myocardial revascularization (ESMR), and therapeutic angiogenesis using protein, gene, or cell therapy. Table 4 lists various non-pharmacological therapies for patients with RA. Of these, only EECP is approved by FDA and is discussed in detail below.

Enhanced external counterpulsation therapy (EECP) is approved by the FDA for the treatment of acute myocardial infarction, cardiogenic shock, congestive heart failure, and stable angina. Approval for the acute MI and cardiogenic shock dates prior to thrombolytic therapy and PCI. Currently, EECP is most commonly applied in the setting of stable angina. However, it is also indicated for patients with class II-III heart failure. EECP was recommended as one of the treatment options for patients with stable angina but was given a class IIb indication in 2002 ACC/AHA guidelines owing to lack of data at that time [40]. Basically, EECP is a non-invasive treatment that involves placing compressible cuffs around the calves and lower and upper thighs. The usual EECP treatment regimen is 35 h administered 1–2 h/day [41] . Contraindications to EECP include: arrhythmias that interfere with the triggering of the EECP system, bleeding diathesis or warfarin therapy with INR ³ 3.0, current or recent (within 2 months) lower extremity thrombophlebitis, severe lower extremity vaso-occlusive disease, severe pulmonary hypertension (pulmonary artery mean pressure>50 mmHg), and presence of a documented aortic aneurysm requiring surgical repair and pregnancy [41]. Uncontrolled HTN, acute decompensated heart failure must be medically optimized and BP controlled prior to initiation of EECP.

Although the precise mechanism of action remains unclear, proposed hypothesis include enhanced diastolic flow, the possible collateralization of coronary vessels and an improvement in endothelial function [42]. The cuffs are inflated sequentially so that during early diastole they cause retrograde blood flow in the aorta, increases coronary artery mean pressure, increased diastolic pressure, and increased venous return [43,44]. When deflated at end of diastole allow the blood vessels to return to their normal state and result in unloading of the left ventricle and decreased systolic blood pressure [44]. The increased cardiac output is related, in part, to increased venous return and augmentation of atrial preload that occurs with EECP [45] .The effectiveness of this intervention for patients with refractory angina has been investigated in a number of international studies over the last 3 decades. Several studies have demonstrated significant improvements in exercise tolerance, time to ST depression during treadmill exercise testing, angina, nitroglycerin use, myocardial perfusion, and quality of life [46-53].

The Multicenter Study of Enhanced External Counterpulsation (MUST-EECP)was a prospective, multicenter, randomized controlled trial to assess the safety and efficacy of EECP in patients with stable angina [48] . Patients we reenrolled in the study if they had class I, II, or III angina; evidence of ischemia on an exercise treadmill test; and documented evidence of coronary artery disease. Patients with revascularization in the preceding 3 months, overt congestive heart failure or a left ventricular ejection fraction ≤30%, significant valvular heart disease, uncontrolled hypertension, permanent pacemaker or implantable cardiac defibrillator, uncontrolled arrhythmias, and significant stenosis of the left main coronary artery without bypass were excluded. Health-related quality of life was assessed at baseline, immediately after EECP and at 1 year. Compared to controls, patients in the active treatment arm had significant increase in time to ≥ 1 mm ST depression and a decrease in the frequency of angina along with significant improvements in all quality of life scales immediately after EECP that persisted at 1 year. However, there was no significant difference in exercise duration or in the amount of sublingual nitroglycerin used in this trial [49].

In summary, EECP results in diastolic augmentation, increased coronary artery perfusion pressure, and decreased left ventricular work. It is associated with improved myocardial perfusion during stress testing, increased levels of nitric oxide and angiogenic growth factors, and improved endothelial function. Clinically, EECP reduces angina by ≥1 CCS class in over 70% of patients and is an attractive, noninvasive, and safe therapeutic intervention for patients with angina who are not optimal candidates for revascularization [50].

Future Directions

Refractory angina is a debilitating condition and its treatment remains problematic. Due to advances in revascularization strategies and medical therapies, the survival of patients with atherosclerotic coronary artery disease has improved substantially over the past two decades. Thegoals of therapy need to be individualized in each case and optimal medical therapy and risk factor modification is the first step for prognostic and symptomatic benefit. A number of promising new pharmacological and non-pharmacological approaches including EECP, TENS and SCS are promising modalities.

References

[1]   Soran O. Treatment options for refractory angina pectoris: Enhanced external counterpulsation therapy. *Curr Treat Options Cardiovasc Med,* 2009; 11: 54–60.
[2]   Kim MC, Kini A, Sharma SK. Refractory angina pectoris: mechanism and therapeutic options. *J Am Coll Cardiol.* 2002 Mar 20;39(6):923-34.
[3]   Ben-Dor I, Battler A. Treatment of stable angina. *Heart.* 2007 Jul;93(7):868-74.
[4]   Mannheimer C, Camici P, Chester MR, et al. The problem of chronic refractory angina; report from the ESC joint study group on the treatmentof refractory angina. *Eur Heart J.* 2002;23(5):355–70.
[5]   Kim MC, Kini A, Sharma SK. Refractory angina pectoris: mechanism and therapeutic options. *J Am Coll Cardiol.* 2002;39(6):923–34.
[6]   Manchanda A, Soran O. Enhanced external counterpulsation and future directions: Step beyond medical management for patients with angina and heart failure. *J Am Coll Cardiol,* 2007; 50: 1523—1531.
[7]   Mukherjee D, Bhatt D, Roe MT, Patel V, Ellis SG. Direct myocardial revascularization and angiogenesis: how many patients might be eligible? *Am J Cardiol* 1999;84:598–600.
[8]   Mannheimer C, Camici P, Chester MR, et al. The proble*m of chronic refractory* angina: report from the ESC Joint Study Group on the Treatment of Refractory Angina. *Eur Heart J.* 2002;23:355–70.

[9] Henry TD, Satran D, Johnson RJ, et al. Natural history of patients with refractory angina. *J Am Coll Cardiol.* 2006;47:231A.

[10] Bache RJ, Dymek DJ. Local and regional regulation of coronary vascular tone. *Prog Cardiovasc Dis.* 1981;24(3):191–212.

[11] Baim DS, Grossman W. *Grossman's cardiac catheterization, angiography, and intervention.* 7th ed. Philadelphia: Lippincott, Williams andWilkins; 2006.

[12] TenVaarwerk IA, Jessurun GA, DeJongste MJ, Andersen C, Mannheimer C, Eliasson T, et al. Clinical outcome of patients treated with spinal cord stimulation for therapeutically refractory angina pectoris. The Working Group on Neurocardiology. *Heart.* 1999;82:82–8.

[13] Abrams J. Clinical practice. Chronic stable angina. *N Engl J Med* 2005;352:2524–33.

[14] Hippisley-Cox J, Coupland C. Effect of combinations of drugs on all cause mortality in patients with ischemic heart disease: nested case-control analysis. *BMJ.* 2005;330(7499):1059–63.

[15] Kjekshus J, Pedersen TR. Reducing the risk of coronary events: evidence from the Scandinavian Simvastatin Survival Study (4S). *Am J Cardiol.* 1995;76(9):64C–8.

[16] Pauly DF, Pepine CJ. Ischemic heart disease: metabolic approaches to management. *Clin Cardiol.* 2004;27(8):439–41.

[17] Khan SN, Dutka DP. A systematic approach to refractory angina. *CurrOpin Support Palliat Care.* 2008;2(4):247–51.

[18] Siddiqui MA, Keam SJ. Ranolazine: a review of its use in chronic stable angina pectoris. *Drugs* 2006;66:693–710.

[19] Chaitman BR, Skettino SL, Parker JO, Hanley P, Meluzin J, Kuch J, et al. Anti-ischemic effects and long-term survival during ranolazine monotherapy in patients with chronic severe angina. *J Am Coll Cardiol.* 2004;43(8):1375–82.

[20] Chaitman BR. Ranolazine for the treatment of chronic angina and potential use in other cardiovascular conditions. *Circulation.* 2006;113(20):2462–72.

[21] Chaitman BR, Pepine CJ, Parker JO, Skopal J, Chumakova G, Kuch J, et al. Effects of ranolazine with atenolol, amlodipine, or diltiazem on exercise tolerance and angina frequency in patients with severe chronic angina: a randomized controlled trial. *JAMA.* 2004;291(3):309–16.

[22] Chazov EI, Lepakchin VK, Zharova EA, et al. Trimetazidine in angina combination therapy – the TACT study: trimetazidine versus conventional treatment in patients with stable angina pectoris in a randomized, placebo-controlled, multicenter study. *Am J Ther.* 2005;12(1):35–42.

[23] Ciapponi A, Pizarro R, Harrison J. Trimetazidine for stable angina. *Cochrane Database Syst Rev* 2005;19:CD003614.(revised 2009)

[24] Ashrafian H, Horowitz JD, Frenneaux MP. Perhexiline. *Cardiovasc Drug Rev.* 2007;25(1):76–97.

[25] Killalea SM, Krum H. Systematic review of the efficacy and safety of perhexiline in the treatment of ischemic heart disease. *Am J Cardiovasc Drugs.* 2001;1(3):193–204.

[26] Markham A, Plosker GL, Goa KL. Nicorandil: an updated review of its use in ischemic heart disease with emphasis on its cardioprotective effects. *Drugs.* 2000;60:955-974.

[27] Ciampricotti R, Schotborgh CE, de Kam PJ, van Herwaarden RH. A comparison of nicorandil with isosorbide mononitrate in elderly patients with stable coronary heart disease: the SNAPE study. *Am Heart J.* 2000;139:939-943.

[28] Di Somma S, Liguori V, Petitto M, et al. A double-blind comparison of nicorandil and metoprolol in stable effort angina pectoris. *Cardiovasc Drugs Ther*. 1993;7:119-123.

[29] Meeter K, Kelder JC, Tijssen JG, et al. Efficacy of nicorandil versus propranolol in mild stable angina pectoris of effort: a long-term, double-blind, randomized study. *J Cardiovasc Pharmacol*. 1992;20(suppl 3):S59-S66.

[30] Raftery EB, Lahiri A, Hughes LO, Rose EL. A double-blind comparison of a beta-blocker and a potassium channel opener in exercise induced angina. *Eur Heart J*. 1993;14(suppl B):35-39.

[31] IONA Study Group. Effect of nicorandil on coronary events in patients with stable angina: the impact of nicorandil in angina (IONA) randomized trial. *Lancet*. 2002;359(9314):1269–75.

[32] Bois P, Bescond J, Renaudon B, Lenfant J. Mode of action of bradycardic agent, S 16257, on ionic currents of rabbit sinoatrial node cells. *Br J Pharmacol*. 1996;118:1051-1057.

[33] Tendera M, Borer JS, Tardif J-C. Effi cacy of I(f) inhibition with ivabradine in different subpopulations with stable angina pectoris. *Cardiology*. 2009;114(2):116–25.

[34] Marquis-Gravel G, Tardif JC. Ivabradine: the evidence of its therapeutic impact in angina. *Core Evid*. 2008;3(1):1–12.

[35] Chou TM, Sudhir K, Hutchison SJ, et al. Testosterone induces dilation of canine coronary conductance and resistance arteries in vivo. *Circulation*. 1996;94:2614-2619.

[36] Yue P, Chatterjee K, Beale C, Poole-Wilson PA, Collins P. Testosterone relaxes rabbit coronary arteries and aorta. *Circulation*. 1995;91:1154-1160.

[37] Magness RR, Rosenfeld CR. Local and systemic estradiol-17 beta: effects on uterine and systemic vasodilation. *Am J Physiol*. 1989;256(4, pt 1):E536-E542.

[38] Thompson LP, Pinkas G, Weiner CP. Chronic 17beta-estradiol replacement increases nitric oxide-mediated vasodilation of guinea pig coronary microcirculation. *Circulation*. 2000;102:445-451.

[39] Hulley S, Grady D, Bush T, et al, Heart and Estrogen/progestin eplacement Study (HERS) Research Group. Randomized trial of estrogen plus progestin for secondary prevention of coronary heart disease in postmenopausal women. *JAMA*. 1998;280:605-613.

[40] Gibbons RJ, Antman EM, Alpert JS et al.ACC/AHA 2002 guideline update for the management of patients with chronic stable angina.*A report of the American College of Cardiology/* American Heart Association Task Force on Pra*ctice* Guidelines (Committee to update the 1999 guidelines for the management of patients with chronic stable angina).Available:http://circ.ahajournals.org/cgi/content/full/107/1/149?maxtoshow=an dHITS=10andhits=10andRESULTFORMAT=andfulltext=guidelines+chronic+stable+a nginaandsearchid=1andFIRSTINDEX=0andresourcetype=HW CIT

[41] Michaels AD, McCullough PA, Soran OZ, et al. Primer: practical approach to the selection of patients for and application of EECP. *NatClin Pract Cardiovasc Med*. 2006; 3(11):623–32.

[42] Cohn PF. Enhanced external counterpulsation for the treatment of angina pectoris. *Progress in Cardiovascular Diseases* 2006;49(2):88–97

[43] Lawson WE, Hui JCK. Enhanced external counterpulsation for chronic myocardial ischemia. *J Crit Illn*. 2000;15(11): 629–36.

[44] Michaels AD, Accad M, Ports TA, Grossman W. Left ventricular systolic unloading and augmentation of intracoronary pressure and Doppler fl ow during enhanced external counterpulsation. *Circulation.* 2002;106(10):1237–42.

[45] Taguchi I, Ogawa K, Kanaya T, Matsuda R, Kuga H, Nakatsugawa M. Effects of enhanced external counterpulsation on hemodynamics and its mechanism. *Circ J.* 2004;68(11):1030–4.

[46] Lawson WE, Hui JC, Soroff HS, et al. Effi cacy of enhanced external counterpulsation in the treatment of angina pectoris. *Am J Cardiol.* 1992;70(9):859–62.

[47] Lawson WE, Hui JC, Zheng ZS, et al. Improved exercise tolerance following enhanced external counterpulsation: cardiac or peripheral effect? *Cardiology.* 1996;87(4):271–5.

[48] Arora RR, Chou TM, Jain D, et al. The multicenter study of enhanced external counterpulsation (MUST-EECP): effect of EECP on exercise-induced myocardial ischemia and anginal episodes. *J Am Coll Cardiol.* 1999;33(7):1833–40.

[49] Arora RR, Chou TM, Jain D, et al. Effects of enhanced external counterpulsation on health-related quality of life continue 12 months after treatment: a substudy of the Multicenter Study of Enhanced External Counterpulsation. *J Investig Med.* 2002;50(1):25–32.

[50] Bart BA. EECP. G.W. Barsness and D.R. Holmes Jr. (eds.), *Coronary Artery Disease,* 2012. Springer-Verlag London Limited 2012. DOI 10.1007/978-1-84628-712-1_6.

[51] Novo G, Bagger JP, Carta R, Koutroulis G, Hall R, Nihoyannopoulos P. Enhanced external counterpulsation for treatment of refractory angina. *J Cardiovasc Med.* 2006; 7(5):335–9.

[52] Springer S, Fife A, Lawson W, et al. Psychosocial effects of enhanced external counterpulsation in the angina patient: a second study. *Psychosomatics.* 2001;42(2):124–32.

[53] Arora RR, Chou TM, Jain D, et al. Effects of enhanced external counterpulsation on health-related quality of life continue 12 months after treatment: a substudy of the Multicenter Study of Enhanced External Counterpulsation. *J Investig Med.* 2002;50(1):25–32.

In: Current Issues in the Management of Stable Ischemic Heart ... ISBN: 978-1-62417-203-8
Editor: Mukesh Singh   © 2013 Nova Science Publishers, Inc.

Chapter IX

Hibernating Myocardium

Shah Tejaskumar[1], and Pinal Modi[2]*

[1]Mount Sinai Hospital, Chicago, IL, US
[2]John H. Stroger Jr. Hospital of Cook County, Chicago, Illinois, US

Abstract

Approximately 50% of patients with coronary artery disease and impaired left ventricular (LV) function have areas of viable myocardium. This can be reversible if myocardial blood supply is reestablished. This viable myocardium is referred to as hibernating myocardium. The exact mechanisms that lead to hibernating myocardium are not known but believed to be due to persistent ischemia or repetitive episodes of ischemia and reperfusion. Regardless of the mechanism, the recovery of LV function after revascularization depends on the severity and extent of ischemic damage and related to the number of dysfunctional but viable segments. Therefore, the identification of dysfunctional myocardial segments with residual viability that can improve after revascularization is pivotal for further patient management. Current evidence indicates that FDG-PET has the highest sensitivity, followed by other nuclear techniques, and dobutamine echocardiography has the lowest sensitivity for detection of hibernating myocardium. Cardiac MRI offers even greater promise of high accuracy in identifying hibernating myocardium. This chapter focuses on evaluation and management of hibernating myocardium.

Background

Chronic left ventricular dysfunction is a sequel of myocardial ischemia manifesting as an impaired cardiac function due to coronary artery disease (CAD). When myocardial ischemia

---

* Correspondent Author: Tejaskumar Shah. 1500 South California Ave, Department of Cardiology, Mount Sinai Hospital, Chicago, IL – 60608. Phone No: 1-551-689-7274. Fax No: 1-773-257-6726. Email: shahtejasm@gmail.com.

is prolonged, it causes myocyte death and results in loss of contractile function and tissue infarction. For many years, this chronic left ventricular dysfunction was thought to be irreversible but recent studies refute this fact and reduced contractile function can be due to stunned myocardium or hibernating myocardium which is reversible after coronary revascularization [1].

The phenomenon of stunned myocardium was first described by Hendricks et al in dogs [2]. Hendricks et al observed that surface electrocardiogram (ECG) findings and regional contraction abnormalities were seen after 5 minutes of occlusion in the left anterior descending coronary artery can be reversible. When the hyperemic response subsided, regional contractile function was still depressed, and regional contractility recovered only after several hours [2]. Additionally, Horn et al and Diamond et al also suggested that inotropic stimulation with epinephrine or dobutamine caused improvement in regional and global left ventricular dysfunction in patients with CAD [3, 4]. This concept indicated that ischemic but noninfarcted myocardium can exist in a state of hibernation without cell death. This finding of a hibernating (or adaptive) process has gotten reorganization in perspective (Rahimtoola et al) of three large multicentre randomized trials of coronary artery bypass surgery for chronic stable angina which is frequently detected in patients with ischemic heart failure and can be reversible after revascularization [5].

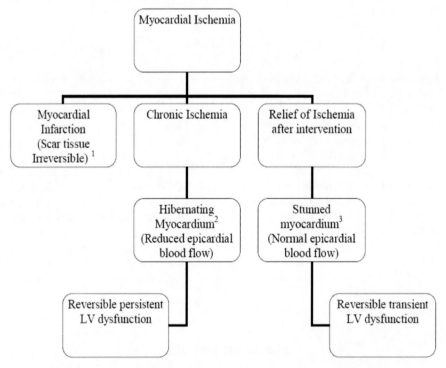

Algorithmic representation of results of chronic ischemia 1) infarction (cell death), 2) chronic ischemia with contractile dysfunction (hibernating myocardium), and 3) transient ischemia (stunned myocardium) with restored blood flow with transient contractile dysfunction.

Figure 1. Consequences of chronic ischemia.

Based on previous observations, there are three potential consequences of chronic ischemia that include myocardial infarction (scar tissue), stunned myocardium (transient post-ischemic dysfunction after reperfusion) and hibernating myocardium (chronic ischemia with dysfunction but viable tissue) [6]. Finding all three entities in the same patient with chronic myocardial dysfunction is not uncommon (Figure 1). Some authors have suggested that stunning and hibernating myocardium represent the processes by which the ischemic myocardium adapts to reduced myocardial oxygen supply to maintain cellular integrity [6]. This chapter focuses on evaluation and management of hibernating myocardium.

Definition and Characteristics of Hibernating Myocardium

Approximately 50% of patients with previous myocardial infarction (MI) may have areas of hibernating tissue mixed with scar tissue, even in the presence of Q waves on the electrocardiogram [7]. Therefore, hibernating myocardium should be suspected in all patients who present with new onset of heart failure or evidence of moderate to severe LV dysfunction in setting of CAD [7].

The extent and severity of ventricular dysfunction can be limited to a discrete portion of ventricle with normal systolic function, or it may involve global impairment of LV function and result in the clinical syndrome of heart failure. In many patients, preexisting collateral vessels and newly developed vessels in the coronary circulation can result in preservation of normal LV function despite the presence of CAD [7]. By and large hibernating myocardium is characterized by the following [7]:

1. Acute and/or chronically reduced blood flow that causes decrease in the myocardial contractile function.
2. Tissue ischemia and resultant remodeling without necrosis, which causes prioritization of metabolic process in the myocardial cell relative to contractile function.
3. Residual contractile reserve in response to inotropic stimulation.
4. Recovery of contractile function after successful revascularization.

Pathophysiology of Myocardial Hibernation

There are two major mechanisms for myocardial stunning. First, post-ischemic dysfunction may be due to cytotoxic oxygen-derived free radicals (i.e., hydroxyl radicals, superoxide anions) that are thought to be generated during occlusion or, upon reperfusion [8, 9]. Second, a calcium overload at the time of reperfusion followed by a partial failure of normal beat-to-beat calcium cycling, occurring at the level of the sarcoplasmic reticulum. These two mechanisms account for transient contractile dysfunction in case of myocardial stunning despite restoration of epicardial blood flow [8, 9]. It is believed that repetitive myocardial stunning results in hibernation. This progression from stunning to hibernation can be fairly short or long, and it depends on the degree of flow impairment in a stenotic coronary artery that supplies the dysfunctional segment. Myocardial hibernation results from a reduction in the coronary perfusion reserve from critical coronary stenosis. Conti et al showed that the production of an acute and critical reduction in coronary flow reserve (CFR) in chronically instrumented pigs leads to an accelerated progression of chronic stunning to hibernation in less than 2 weeks [10, 11].

Ischemic threshold progressively decreases with reduction in CFR, and, repetitive stunning leads to a delay in the recovery of function that lasts longer than the interval between ischemic episodes [6]. Hibernation in a patient with severe fixed coronary stenosis is more likely because coronary flow will fluctuate continuously due to combination of severe epicardial stenosis and loss of local auto regulation [6]. Thus, myocardium may down regulate its function to a low level to achieve a metabolic balance between demand and supply. In many situations (e.g., exercise, stress, patient with a history of unstable angina), this balance may be continuously upset by recurrent reduction of flow followed by stunning. In these situations, a deficit in function results from a complex combination of hibernation, ischemic dysfunction, and stunning [6]. Chronic repetitive ischemia or stunning that progress to hibernation is associated with regional down regulation of the sarcoplasmic reticulum, with changes in calcium regulation and gene expression [8, 9].

These changes are accompanied by modest increases in myocyte apoptosis and a reduction in the regional myocyte nuclear density. These same structural and functional findings occur in patients with dilated cardiomyopathy of ischemic origin.

Pathologic Findings

Histological specimens obtained at the time of surgery demonstrate profound structural changes in dysfunctional but viable myocardium. These changes include progressive loss of contractile proteins in sarcomere without loss of cell volume. Depletion of sarcomere near the perinuclear region may extend to the entire cell and numerous small mitochondria can be found in the areas adjacent to the glycogen-rich perinuclear zone [12]. In addition to substantial loss of sarcoplasmic reticulum, there is loss and disorganization of T-tubules [12].

Evaluation of Hibernating Myocardium

Hibernating myocardium is viable, and this viability can be determined with a variety of imaging techniques that depict either the contractility of myocardial tissue when stimulated or the persistence of metabolic activity within the region of dysfunctional myocardium. The following modalities can be used to distinguish between myocardium with potential for improvement in function and myocardium that does not improve after revascularization.

1. SPECT imaging (Single Photon Emission Computed Tomography): ^{201} Thallium scintigraphy, ^{99m} Tc-sestamibi (MIBI), ^{99m} Tc-tetrafosmin
2. PET imaging: ^{82} Rb, ^{13} NH$_3$, ^{18} FDG, ^{14} C-acetate

3. Dobutamine or exercise echocardiography: Assessment of regional function.
4. MRI imaging: To assess regional perfusion and wall function.

1. SPECT Imaging

Thallium Scintigraphy

Myocardial retention of the potassium analog [201] Thallium can be detected by using single photon emission computed tomography (SPECT). Normal thallium uptakes with exercise and thallium defects that redistribute on images obtained after a 3-4-hour delay are accurate predictors of viable myocardium. However, the absence or lack of thallium uptake does not necessarily indicate myocardial scarring, because severely ischemic but viable myocardium, as well as a mixture of scar and viable myocardium, may also produce an "irreversible defect" [12].

Segments that are likely to improve have thallium activity that is more than 50% of the activity of healthy myocardium. From 45-75% of persistent early defects exhibit normal perfusion after revascularization. In these cases, standard redistribution images obtained after 3-4 hours may not help in the differentiation of hibernating myocardium from scarred myocardium and reinjection or 24-hour thallium protocol may reduce the false assessment of irreversible defect present after 3-4 hours [13].

In hibernating myocardium, the initial uptake is low but then increases gradually. This phenomenon is related to [201] Thallium redistribution. Regional thallium activity on early (at 3-4 h) or late (at 8-72 h) redistribution imaging obtained after stress has been used to demonstrate the distribution of viable myocardial cells and the extent of myocardial fibrosis. A possible explanation for late redistribution (8-72 hours) may be that the initial uptake of thallium during exercise is sufficiently reduced in certain ischemic myocardial regions so that it continues to mimic the appearance of scarred myocardium on early 3-4 hour images [14]. Therefore, if more time is allowed for redistribution, more viable segments are distinguished from scarred or fibrotic myocardium. Late thallium redistribution, when present, is an accurate indicator of viable myocardium [14].

Reinjection of additional thallium immediately after conventional 3-4 hour imaging significantly improves the detection of viable myocardium in 31-49% of the regions that were interpreted as having an irreversible perfusion defect on conventional redistribution images. Current evidence indicates that the thallium reinjection in otherwise irreversible defects can be used to predict improvement in regional function after revascularization, with a PPV of 80-87% and an NPV of 82-100%. Moreover, thallium reinjection improves the detection of viable myocardium, as shown in several studies, even when regional quantitative analysis is used [13, 15].

Ragosta et al were the first to report that thallium perfusion defects may occur on resting images in patients with CAD in the absence of acute ischemic process or previous myocardial infarction [16]. Available data suggest that rest-redistribution thallium imaging depicts viable myocardium in most reversible regions, but it may cause underestimation of viable myocardium in as much as two thirds of the irreversible regions [16]. In nutshell, thallium scintigraphy involves stress early redistribution imaging, late redistribution imaging at 8-24 hours, reinjection imaging, and rest redistribution imaging [16].

Role of ^{99m} Tc-MIBI SPECT

The ^{99m} Tc-MIBI is only minimally redistributed, and it is not taken up by necrotic myocardium. It has a shorter half-life (half-life, 6 hours) than that of thallium (half-life, 2.8 days). Therefore, some have suggested that the use of ^{99m} Tc-MIBI causes underestimation of the viable myocardium. However, when resting myocardial perfusion scintigraphy with ^{99m} Tc-MIBI is combined with administration of nitroglycerin, it may be as effective as redistribution with ^{201} Thallium [17].

The prediction of functional recovery is based on the semi-quantitative analysis of residual MIBI uptake in dysfunctional segments compared with remote areas of high uptake. An uptake of 50-60% is used as the threshold for viable tissue. Similarly, low-dose dobutamine infusion with ^{99m} Tc-MIBI SPECT has been shown to provide better accuracy for predicting functional recovery than rest SPECT [17].

2. PET Imaging

PET is often considered the gold standard for the detection of viable myocardium. The mechanism of PET imaging is based on the concept of regional substrate utilization shifts from free fatty acids to glucose in case of ischemic dysfunction and hibernating myocardium [18]. Schwaiger et al showed that in patients with advanced CAD, production of the glucose protein transporter (GLUT) protein is increased as is the expression of myocardial glucose transporter messenger RNA protein [12]. FDG (fluorodeoxyglucose) is a glucose analogue that is intracellularly phosphorylated to FDG-6-phosphate in the myocardium. An increased uptake of ^{18} FDG in relation to perfusion or flow-metabolism mismatch is indicative of hibernating myocardium, whereas matched defects are indicative of scar tissue; values in between these represent healthy myocardial tissue mixed with fibrosis [19].

Compared with thallium-SPECT imaging, FDG-PET imaging provides better results for the differentiation of viable myocardium from scarred myocardium. Brunken et al published data from a comparison of tomographic thallium images with PET images; 47% of the irreversible thallium defects were identified as viable on PET images [20]. The predictive accuracy achieved with PET images is comparable to that of thallium images, with a positive predictive value (PPV) of 80-87% and a negative predictive value (NPV) of 82-100%. Tamaki et al subsequently confirmed these findings in two comparative studies of SPECT and PET in which 38-42% of the irreversible thallium defects had enhanced with FDG uptake suggestive of viable myocardium [21]. Thus, conventional stress-redistribution ^{201} Thallium imaging has a low predictive value in the identification of viable myocardium when compared with PET.

3. Dobutamine Echocardiography

Newer data of complete protocol (i.e. low and high dose) dobutamine echocardiography show an improved survival after revascularization if at least four viable dys-synergic LV segments in a 16 segment model can be identified. This protocol can elicit several types of contractile responses (sustained improvement in contraction or monophasic response, biphasic response, new wall motion abnormality) which should be interpreted in view of other clinical data including a previous infarction. The test protocol can be used safely at the end of the first week after myocardial infarction [22, 23]. This technique uses a progressively increasing dose of dobutamine, which first augments regional function and then induces ischemic wall motion abnormalities by increasing the myocardial oxygen demand in the presence of coronary stenosis.

Pre- interventional identification of improved systolic wall thickening with inotropic stimulation (low-dose dobutamine - 5 to 10mcg/kg/minute) at echocardiography has been a preferred method. Viable myocardial segments thicken in response to dobutamine. With increasing doses of dobutamine, up to 40 mcg/kg/minute, deterioration of functional wall thickening occurs, and akinesis and lack of synergy result in the so-called biphasic response [22, 23].

Several authors have shown that the biphasic response during dobutamine infusion is best predictor of improvement [22, 23, and 24]. This has a PPV (positive predictive value) of 83% and an NPV of 81% for improvement after revascularization.

4. Cardiac MRI

Because of the noninvasive nature of MRI, cine MRI (cMRI) of the heart is an excellent method for the assessment of regional wall motion. Baer and coworkers reported findings in 35 patients with myocardial infarction and regional akinesis or dyskinesis who underwent rest and dobutamine MRI as well as FDG analysis [25]. Recently, diagnostic accuracy of cardiac magnetic resonance (CMR) assessing myocardial viability in patients with chronic left ventricular (LV) dysfunction due to coronary artery disease using 3 techniques: 1) end-diastolic wall thickness (EDWT); 2) low-dose dobutamine (LDD); and 3) contrast delayed enhancement (DE) has been evaluated. Both the likelihood and the time course of long-term functional improvement are related to the baseline amount of scar, as visualized by CMR [26, 27]. Romero J et al in a meta-analysis of 24 studies investigated the role of CMR in evaluating myocardial viability using 3 different techniques and they found that DE-CMR provides the highest sensitivity and NPV, whereas LDD CMR provides the best specificity and PPV [28].

Pearlman et al used a porcine model to measure wall motion and wall thickening during the cardiac cycle [29]. The serial motion assessment by reference tracking (SMART) measurements of wall thickening and motion detects much smaller thickening and motion in ischemic myocardium than fixed radial metrics. It is twice as sensitive in detecting abnormalities of wall motion and thickening and is, thus, useful in differentiating ischemic myocardium from normal myocardium. However further studies are needed to validate the system for clinical evaluation [29].

Bax et al performed a meta-analysis of various perfusion imaging and echocardiography techniques and their usefulness in the prediction of myocardial viability (Table 1) [30, 31]. The data revealed that the sensitivity in predicting improved regional contractile function after revascularization was high for all techniques analyzed; however, specificity varied greatly and was lowest for[201] Thallium stress-redistribution and[201] Thallium rest-redistribution imaging. Specificity was highest for low-dose dobutamine echocardiography. Other data suggested that dobutamine MRI with SMART (serial motion assessment reference tracking) tagging and/or point trajectory assessment is the most accurate because it has better endocardial definition, has higher resolution, and corrects for tethering. It is still evolving and not widely available. The negative predictive value was highest for MRI or FDG PET [29, 30, and 31].

Table 1. Sensitivity and Specificity of Different Methods in the Detection of Hibernating Myocardium in Different Studies [6, 30 and 31]

Test	Sensitivity, % *	Specificity, % *	No. of Patients
MIBI	83 (78-87)	69 (63-74)	207
Dobutamine echocardiography	84 (82-86)	81 (79-84)	448
[201] Tl reinjection	86 (86-89)	47 (43-51)	209
FDG PET	88 (84-91)	73 (69-74)	332
[201] Tl rest-redistribution	90 (87-93)	54 (49-60)	145

* Data in parentheses are ranges.
** Sensitivity is defined as the number of viable segments of myocardium divided by the number with recovery of function. Specificity is defined as the number of nonviable segments divided by the number without recovery of function. Values for sensitivity and specificity are weighted means. There are no significant differences in sensitivity among the techniques. Both thallium-201 tests have significantly less specificity than the other methods; dobutamine echocardiography has greater specificity than the other methods. Data are from Bax et al. [6, 30, and 31].

Treatment and Prognosis

Patients with CAD are often referred for revascularization because of angina or chronic ventricular dysfunction with viable myocardium. The most important benefit of this procedure is improvement of the global ejection fraction [6]. This improvement is directly related to the number of dysfunctional but viable segments. This is more obvious when functional response to exercise or dobutamine infusion is evaluated after treatment. The magnitude of improvement in the symptoms of heart failure and in exercise capacity is proportional to the mass of revascularized myocardium that was demonstrated to be viable before revascularization [6].

The results of the Coronary Artery Surgery Study (CASS), in which bypass surgery was compared with medical treatment, indicate that patients with multi vessel disease and LV dysfunction benefited most from surgery in terms of survival. Revascularization improves the prognosis of patients with hibernating myocardium. Therefore, the identification of patients with hibernating myocardium is vital to overall treatment of patients with CAD [6, 32].

The evaluation before revascularization in patients with LV dysfunction includes the following:

- Assess the presence of available target vessels for bypass or angioplasty.
- Consider other risk factors for death after bypass surgery (e.g., age, sex, comorbid condition, prior surgery, valvular diseases).

- Consider hemodynamic support during angioplasty (use of an intra-aortic balloon pump or percutaneous circulatory assistance).
- Evaluate the extent of viable myocardium in the distribution of the target vessels.
- If severe heart failure is present, consider use of a device to assist the LV or cardiac transplantation [6, 32].

Recently, the Surgical Treatment for Ischemic Heart Failure (STICH) trial, a randomized comparison of coronary artery bypass graft (CABG) surgery and medical therapy alone in 1212 patients with CAD amenable to CABG with a left ventricular ejection fraction under 35% were published. The primary end point was all-cause death. There was no significant difference between medical therapy alone and medical therapy plus CABG with respect to the primary end point of death from any cause. Patients assigned to CABG, as compared with those assigned to medical therapy alone, had lower rates of death from cardiovascular causes and of death from any cause or hospitalization for cardiovascular causes [33]. Another study [33], a randomized comparison of medical therapy with or without bypass surgery for ischemic heart disease in patients with LV systolic dysfunction based on myocardial viability, found that: overall, substantial viable myocardium evident at baseline imaging studies had no independent bearing on all-cause mortality over five years; and as such viability didn't influence the relative effectiveness of the two treatment strategies, either for all-cause mortality or the secondary end points of CV mortality and CV hospitalization[34]. However, this study had several limitations including lack of randomization and limited power in both subgroup along with method of assessment of viability (SPECT imaging and dobutamine echocardiography). As techniques evolved, many new evidences regarding cardiac MR (CMR) are emerging for its ability to predict myocardial viability and revascularization lead LV function recovery [35].

References

[1]   Ferrari R, Ceconi C, Curello S, Benigno M, La Canna G, Visioli O. Left ventricular dysfunction due to the new ischemic outcomes: stunning and hibernation. *J. Cardiovasc. Pharmacol.* 1996;28 Suppl 1:S18-26.

[2]   Heyndrickx GR, Millard RW, McRitchie RJ, Maroko PR, Vatner SF. Regional myocardial functional and electrophysiological alterations after brief coronary artery occlusion in conscious dogs. *J. Clin. Invest. Oct.* 1975; 56(4):978-85.

[3]   Horn HR, Teichholz LE, Cohn PF, Herman MV, Gorlin R. Augmentation of left ventricular contraction pattern in coronary artery disease by an inotropic catecholamine: the epinephrine ventriculogram. *Circulation* 1974;49:1063-71.

[4]   Diamond GA, Forrester JS, deLuz PL, Wyatt HL, Swan HJC. Post-extrasystolic potentiation of ischemic myocardium by atrial stimulation. *Am. Heart J.* 1978;95: 204-9.

[5]   Rahimtoola SH. A perspective on the three large multicenter randomized clinical trials of coronary bypass surgery for chronic stable angina. *Circulation* 1985; Suppl V:72:V-123–V-135.

[6] William Wijns, M.D., Stephen F. Vatner, M.D., and Paolo G. Camici, M.D. Hibernating Myocardium. *N. Engl. J. Med.* 1998; 339:173-181.

[7] Cooper HA, Braunwald E. Clinical importance of stunned and hibernating myocardium. *Coron Artery Dis.* Aug 2001;12(5):387-92.

[8] Bolli R. Mechanism of myocardial "stunning". *Circulation.* Sep 1990; 82(3):723-38.

[9] Bolli R. Oxygen-derived free radicals and myocardial reperfusion injury: an overview. *Cardiovasc. Drugs Ther.* Mar 1991;5 Suppl 2:249-68.

[10] Conti CR. The stunned and hibernating myocardium: a brief review. *Clin. Cardiol.* Sep 1991;14(9):708-12.

[11] Laky D, Parascan L. Hibernating myocardium, morphological studies on intraoperatory myocardial biopsies and on chronic ischemia experimental model. *Rom. J. Morphol. Embryol.* 2007;48(4):407-13.

[12] Gibson RS, Watson DD, Taylor GJ, Crosby IK, Wellons HL, Holt ND. Prospective assessment of regional myocardial perfusion before and after coronary revascularization surgery by quantitative thallium-201 scintigraphy. *J. Am. Coll. Cardiol.* Mar 1983;1(3):804-15.

[13] Dilsizian V, Freedman NM, Bacharach SL, Perrone-Filardi P, Bonow RO. Regional thallium uptake in irreversible defects. Magnitude of change in thallium activity after reinjection distinguishes viable from nonviable myocardium. *Circulation.* Feb 1992; 85(2):627-34.

[14] Camici P, Ferrannini E, Opie LH. Myocardial metabolism in ischemic heart disease: basic principles and application to imaging by positron emission tomography. *Prog. Cardiovasc. Dis.* Nov-Dec 1989;32(3):217-38.

[15] Sun D, Nguyen N, DeGrado TR, Schwaiger M, Brosius FC 3rd. Ischemia induces translocation of the insulin-responsive glucose transporter GLUT4 to the plasma membrane of cardiac myocytes. *Circulation.* Feb 1994;89(2):793-8.

[16] Brunken RC, Mody FV, Hawkins RA, Nienaber C, Phelps ME, Schelbert HR. Positron emission tomography detects metabolic viability in myocardium with persistent 24-hour single-photon emission computed tomography 201Tl defects. *Circulation.* Nov 1992; 86(5):1357-69.

[17] Tamaki N, Ohtani H, Yamashita K, Magata Y, Yonekura Y, Nohara R. Metabolic activity in the areas of new fill-in after thallium-201 reinjection: comparison with positron emission tomography using fluorine-18-deoxyglucose. *J. Nucl. Med.* Apr 1991; 32(4):673-8.

[18] Kayden DS, Sigal S, Soufer R, Mattera J, Zaret BL, Wackers FJ. Thallium-201 for assessment of myocardial viability: quantitative comparison of 24-hour redistribution imaging with imaging after reinjection at rest. *J. Am. Coll. Cardiol.* Nov 15 1991; 18(6):1480-6.

[19] Iskandrian AS, Hakki AH, Kane SA, Goel IP, Mundth ED, Hakki AH. Rest and redistribution thallium-201 myocardial scintigraphy to predict improvement in left ventricular function after coronary arterial bypass grafting. *Am. J. Cardiol.* May 1 1983; 51(8):1312-6.

[20] Ragosta M, Beller GA, Watson DD, Kaul S, Gimple LW. Quantitative planar rest-redistribution 201Tl imaging in detection of myocardial viability and prediction of improvement in left ventricular function after coronary bypass surgery in patients with severely depressed left ventricular function. *Circulation.* May 1993;87(5):1630-41.

[21] Cigarroa CG, deFilippi CR, Brickner ME, Alvarez LG, Wait MA, Grayburn PA. Dobutamine stress echocardiography identifies hibernating myocardium and predicts recovery of left ventricular function after coronary revascularization. *Circulation.* Aug 1993; 88(2): 430-6.

[22] Perrone-Filardi P, Pace L, Prastaro M, Piscione F, Betocchi S, Squame F. Dobutamine echocardiography predicts improvement of hypoperfused dysfunctional myocardium after revascularization in patients with coronary artery disease. *Circulation.* May 15 1995; 91(10):2556-65.

[23] Afridi I, Kleiman NS, Raizner AE, Zoghbi WA. Dobutamine echocardiography in myocardial hibernation. Optimal dose and accuracy in predicting recovery of ventricular function after coronary angioplasty. *Circulation.* Feb 1 1995;91(3):663-70.

[24] Bisi G, Sciagrà R, Santoro GM, Fazzini PF. Rest technetium-99m sestamibi tomography in combination with short-term administration of nitrates: feasibility and reliability for prediction of postrevascularization outcome of asynergic territories. *J. Am. Coll. Cardiol.* Nov 1 1994; 24(5): 1282-9.

[25] Baer FM, Voth E, Schneider CA, et al. Comparison of low-dose dobutamine-gradient-echo magnetic resonance imaging and positron emission tomography with [18F]fluorodeoxyglucose in patients with chronic coronary artery disease. A functional and morphological approach to the detection of residua. *Circulation.* 1995/02; 91(4): 1006-15.

[26] Kim RJ, Wu E, Rafael A, Chen EL, Parker MA, Simonetti O. The use of contrast-enhanced magnetic resonance imaging to identify reversible myocardial dysfunction. *N. Engl. J. Med.* Nov 16 2000;343(20):1445-53.

[27] Bondarenko O, Beek AM, Twisk JW, Visser CA, van Rossum AC. Time course of functional recovery after revascularization of hibernating myocardium: a contrast-enhanced cardiovascular magnetic resonance study. *Eur. Heart J.* Jun 13 2008.

[28] Romero J, Xue X, Gonzalez W, Garcia MJ. CMR Imaging Assessing Viability in Patients With Chronic Ventricular Dysfunction Due to Coronary Artery Disease: A Meta-Analysis of Prospective Trials. JACC *Cardiovasc. Imaging.* 2012 May; 5(5): 494-508.

[29] Pearlman JD, Gertz ZM, Wu Y, Simons M, Post MJ. Serial motion assessment by reference tracking (SMART): application to detection of local functional impact of chronic myocardial ischemia. *J. Comput. Assist. Tomogr.* 2001 Jul-Aug;25(4):558-62.

[30] Bax JJ, Wijns W, Cornel JH, Visser FC, Boersma E, Fioretti PM. Accuracy of currently available techniques for prediction of functional recovery after revascularization in patients with left ventricular dysfunction due to chronic coronary artery disease: comparison of pooled data. *J. Am. Coll. Cardiol.* 1997;30:1451-60.

[31] Bax JJ, Cornel JH, Visser FC, Fioretti PM, van Lingen A, Reijs AE. Prediction of recovery of myocardial dysfunction after revascularization. Comparison of fluorine-18 fluorodeoxyglucose/thallium-201 SPECT, thallium-201 stress-reinjection SPECT and dobutamine echocardiography. *J. Am. Coll. Cardiol.* Sep 1996;28(3):558-64.

[32] Caracciolo EA, Davis KB, Sopko G, Kaiser GC, Corley SD, Schaff H, Taylor HA, Chaitman BR. Comparison of surgical and medical group survival in patients with left main coronary artery disease. Long-term CASS experience. *Circulation.* 1995 May 1;91(9):2325-34.

[33] Velazquez EJ, Lee KL, Deja MA, Jain A, Sopko G, Marchenko A, Ali IS, Pohost G, Gradinac S, Abraham WT, Yii M, Prabhakaran D, Szwed H, Ferrazzi P, Petrie MC, O'Connor CM, Panchavinnin P, She L, Bonow RO, Rankin GR, Jones RH, Rouleau JL; STICH Investigators. Coronary-artery bypass surgery in patients with left ventricular dysfunction. *N. Engl. J. Med.* 2011 Apr 28;364(17):1607-16. Epub 2011 Apr 4.

[34] Bonow RO, Maurer G, Lee KL, Holly TA, Binkley PF, Desvigne-Nickens P, Drozdz J, Farsky PS, Feldman AM, Doenst T, Michler RE, Berman DS, Nicolau JC,Pellikka PA, Wrobel K, Alotti N, Asch FM, Favaloro LE, She L, Velazquez EJ, Jones RH, Panza JA; STICH Trial Investigators. Myocardial viability and survival in ischemic left ventricular dysfunction. *N. Engl. J. Med.* 2011 Apr 28;364(17):1617-25. Epub 2011 Apr 4.

[35] Gerber BL, Rousseau MF, Ahn SA, le Polain de Waroux JB, Pouleur AC, Phlips T, Vancraeynest D, Pasquet A, Vanoverschelde JL. Prognostic value of myocardial viability by delayed-enhanced magnetic resonance in patients withcoronary artery disease and low ejection fraction: impact of revascularization therapy. *J. Am. Coll. Cardiol.* 2012 Feb 28;59(9):825-35.

In: Current Issues in the Management of Stable Ischemic Heart ... ISBN: 978-1-62417-203-8
Editor: Mukesh Singh © 2013 Nova Science Publishers, Inc.

Chapter X

Arrhythmia Following Cardiac Surgery

*Abdul Aleem[1], Ravi V. Desai[2] and Nasir Shariff[*2]*
[1] Sri Siddhartha Medical College, Karnataka, India
[2] Lehigh Valley Hospital and Health Network, Allentown, Pennsylvania, US

Abstract

Chronic stable angina is a common medical condition requiring cardiac surgery. Cardiac arrhythmias following cardiac surgery are common and are associated with higher morbidity and mortality. Several factors have been identified to predispose the development of these arrhythmias. The present chapter will address the common and uncommon cardiac arrhythmias following surgery with detailed reference on preventive and management strategies of atrial tachyarrhythmias.

Introduction

Chronic stable angina affects more than 6 million Americans (Gibbons, Chatterjee et al. 1999). Coronary artery bypass surgery is recommended for patients with triple-vessel disease, in particular those with reduced left ventricular ejection fraction (Eagle, Guyton et al. 1999). Cardiac surgery is also performed in patients with significant valve disease or congenital heart diseases. More than 250,000 patients undergo cardiac surgery every year in the United States (Rosamond, Flegal et al. 2008). Cardiac arrhythmias are frequent following surgery in these patients. These arrhythmias could be either in the form of tachy- or brady-arrhythmias. Most arrhythmias following surgery are considered transient and benign while others are associated with increased hospital stay, and worse outcomes. In the present chapter we will focus on the common post operative arrhythmias and their management including prophylactic measures to improve the outcome following surgery.

---

[*] Address for correspondence: Nasir Shariff, MD, Department of Cardiology, Lehigh Valley Hospital and Health Network, Allentown, PA. US, Email: nasirshariff@gmail.com

Atrial Tachyarrhythmia

Atrial fibrillation, flutter, and tachycardia are different forms of atrial tachyarrhythmia that usually coexist in patients after cardiothoracic surgery. They have similar clinical and therapeutic implications and hence are dealt as a single group. They commonly occur early following cardiothoracic surgery with peak incidence during the first 2 to 3 days after surgery. Although these arrhythmias were initially thought of as transient and benign, they have been associated with a two-fold increase in cardiovascular morbidity and mortality. The reported incidences of these arrhythmias are dependent on the patient profile, surveillence method and type of surgery. They occur in about 11 to 40 percent of patients after coronary-artery bypass grafting and in over 50 percent after valvular surgery (Ommen, Odell et al. 1997). The incidence is the highest (>60%) in patients undergoing mitral valve replacement with bypass surgery. There is noted higher occurrence of heart failure and cerebral ischemic accident, both resulting in longer hospital stay, and consequently in higher surgery costs. Atrial fibrillation is associated with longer stay in the intensive care unit of average of 13 hrs and longer hospital stay of 3 days in comparision to patients without this complication after surgery (Mathew, Parks et al. 1996). It is estimated that the hospital charges are $10,000 to $11,000 more per patient with post operative AF (Aranki, Shaw et al. 1996). In a study by Lehey et al atrial fibrillation was the most common diagnosis for patients readmitted within 30 days of discharge after cardiac surgery (Lahey, Campos et al. 1998). Similar to non-surgical atrial fibrillation, post operative arrhythmia is likely associated with left atrial thrombus formation within early period of the event which predisposes these patients to risk of stroke.

Etiology

Atrial flutter/fibrillation is usually attributed to reentry of multiple wavelets of excitation circulating throughout the atria. The exact etiology and electrophysiology of postoperative atrial arrhythmia is not well defined. Atrial premature beats may trigger the occurence of these rhythms in patient with underlying predisposing substrate. Disparity in the atrial conduction periods and refractory periods as occurs with dilated atrial could increase the risk of this problem. These disparities could also occur in situations like atrial ischemia during surgery and following incision of the atrial wall. Recent studies suggest that a multi-factorial mechanism is involved which includes oxidative stress, inflammation, atrial fibrosis, excessive production of catecholamines, changes in autonomic tonus and in the expression of connexins. These changes result in an increase of atrial refractive index dispersion and in the formation of a pro-arrhythmic substrate.

Predisposing Factors

There have been several factors which been identified to predispose to these arrhythmias after cardiac surgery (Table 1). Age and previous history of atrial fibrillation are the two most consistent predisposing factors.

Table 1. Risk factors associated with atrial fibrillation following cardiac surgery

• Pre-operative risk factors
− Advanced age
− Male gender
− Hypertension
− Congestive heart failure
− Chronic obstructive pulmonary disease
− Prior history of atrial fibrillation
− Previous cardiac surgery
− Left ventricular hypertrophy
− Left atrial enlargement
− Holding off beta-blocker or ACE-inhibitors
− Obesity
• Intra-operative risk factors
− Cardiopulmonary bypass time
− Bicaval canulation
− Type of cardiac surgery
− Systemic hypothermia
• Post-operative risk factors
− Post operative infections
− Prolonged ventilation
− Red cell transfusion
− Use of NSAIDs/steroids (negative association)

It is noted that every year increase in age is associated with 1.02 odds ratio increase in chances of atrial fibrillation. Age related changes in the atria such as dilatation, muscle atrophy, and decreased conduction could explain the association. Other factors associated with occurrence of post operative atrial fibrillation include left atrial size, left ventricular wall thickness, signal averaged P wave on ECG, concomitant valvular surgery. Postoperative administration of beta-blockers (OR, 0.32), ACE inhibitors (OR, 0.62), potassium supplementation (OR, 0.53), and nonsteroidal anti-inflammatory drugs (OR, 0.49) have been associated with reduced incidence of these arrhythmias but the results have not been consistent. There has been a noted trend towards reduction of post operative atrial fibrillation with use of angiotensin receptor blockers. Technical advances in surgery and anesthesia have not decreased the incidence of postoperative atrial tachyarrhythmias. Studies have not found different rates of postoperative atrial tachyarrhythmias to be associated with the various cardiac surgical techniques including intermittent aortic cross clamping and hypothermic cardioplegia.

Preventive Strategies

There have been several studies looking at preventive strategies to reduce the occurrences of these arrhythmias considering their high incidence and their association with increased cost of hospitalization and worsened outcome in patients. The most studied medications and their role is discussed further.

Beta Blockers: Beta-blockers act by inhibiting the catecholamine induced electro-physiologic changes in the myocardial cells. These are the most commonly used prophylactic medications to prevent post operative atrial fibrillation (POAF). The benefits of the medications is seen in both patients whose medications were begun prior to surgery and also when the medications were started immediately after surgery. The effect of prevent of POAF has been noted to be independent of the type of beta-blocker used. In a meta-analysis of 27 randomized studies - β-blockers reduced the incidence of POAF by 14% (P<0.00001). The odd ratio of occurrence of AF after surgery in patients receiving the medication varied from 0.01 to 1.34. The cumulative odds ratio was 0.39 (Crystal, Connolly et al. 2002).

Amiodarone: Amiodarone has been shown in several studies to reduce the occurrence of POAF in cardiac surgery patients. In a meta-analysis of 9 studies there was noted reduction in the occurence of AF from 37% in the control group to 22.5% in amiodarone group (OR, 0.48; 95% CI, 0.37 to 0.61) (Crystal, Connolly et al. 2002). (Crystal E. Circ 2002). In a study comparing intravenous infusion of metoprolol to intravenous amiodarone therapy after cardiac surgery – there was similar occurence of AF between the two groups (Halonen, Loponen et al. 2010). In a meta-analysis of the common interventions to reduce POAF, only amiodarone was associated with significantly reduced length of stay, average -0.60 days. It was also the only medication associated with significantly reduced stroke rate (Burgess, Kilborn et al. 2006). For patients who are undergoing elective surgery, amiodarone loading should be started preoperatively whereas for those undergoing emergency surgery, amiodarone could be initiated in the postoperative period. Oral amiodarone at dose of 600mg per day for 7 days before surgery and 200mg per day until the day of discharge form hospital reduced the incidence of post-CABG AF by 45% (25% in treated patients vs. 53% in patients on placebo) (Daoud, Strickberger et al. 1997).

Sotalol: Sotalol has both Class III anti-arrhthymic and beta-blocker properties. It inhibits the potassium channels and can cause prolongation of the QT interval. The incidence of POAF was observed to be 17% in patients receiving sotalol, compared to 37% among patients treated with a placebo. Sotalol has been shown to reduce AF more than other beta-blockers though this did not reach statistically significant numbers. In a meta-analysis of 4 studies, there was noted occurrence of POAF in 12% of patients on sotalol compared to 22% in patients on beta-blockers (OR, 0.50; 95% CI, 0.34 to 0.74) (Patel, Gillinov et al. 2008). Several of the trials used Sotalol pre-operatively 120mg per day continuing post-operatively, and this regimen were not associated with an increase in side effects.

Other preventive strategies: Several other medical interventions have been tried to prevent POAF. Some of the strategies which have been shown to reduce the incidence include atrial pacing after surgery, statins, nitroprusside, N-acetyl cystein, magnesium, steroids and non-steroidal anti-inflammatory medications. Prophylactic overdrive atrial pacing decreases the incidence of POAF by two-thirds. This continuous atrial overdrive pacing was done with epicardial wires in the study (Blommaert, Gonzalez et al. 2000). Effectiveness of nitropruside in reduction of POAF was proven in only one study. In this study, intravenous nitroprusside drip (0.5 microgm/kg/min) in the rewarming period was associated with significant reduction in incidence of POAF (12% vs. 27%) (Cavolli, Kaya et al. 2008). Low magnesium concentrations are independent risk factors of AF after cardiovascular surgery. Magnesium supplement during the perioperative period was shown in a meta-analysis to significantly reduce the incidence of POAF. The largest effect of Mg is in patient who are not on beta-blockers (OR 0.05) (Burgess, Kilborn et al. 2006). Statins have shown inconsitent results on occurence of POAF. Steroids and NSAIDs have been shown to reduce the incidence of POAF but there is concerns regarding adverse effects. Recommendation for prevention: The ACC/AHA/ESC issued guidelines for management of post operative AF in 2006 (Fuster, Ryden et al. 2006). Beta-blockers are recommended as a Class I indication for prevention of POAF. Starting Amiodarone is appropriate for prophylaxis for patients with high risk of POAF (Class IIa recommendation). Prophylaxis with sotalol needs to be considering in patients with high risk of developing AF (Class IIb). Table 2 has the commonly used doses of medications for prophylaxis.

Management

Patients who are hemodynamically unstable with POAF need to be considered for direct current cardioversion. 200 J biphasic waveform current has a very high success rate in conversion (>95%). In a recently published randomized double blinded study Vernakalant a inward ultrarapid potassium current inhibitor was used for chemical cardioversion. A 10-minute infusion of 3 mg/kg vernakalant followed by repeat dose after 15-minutes if not converted was successful in 47% of patients. There was noted sustained effect of the medication with reduced re-occurrences for 24 hours (Kowey, Dorian et al. 2009).

In patients who are hemodynamically stable, issues that need to be addressing comprise of hypoxemia, anemia, hypovolemia and pain control. Nodal blocking agents useful to control heart rate include beta-blockers, calcium channel blockers, digoxin and amiodarone. Metoprolol can be given as intravenous boluses of 2.5 to 5 mg every 5 minutes. Esmolol has a shorter action period and can be given as infusion. Calcium channel blockers which can be given intravenously include diltiazem and verapamil. In patients who have issues of lowish blood pressures; digoxin at the dose of 0.25 mg every 4 hours for 3 to 4 doses could be considered. Amiodarone is also helpful in heart rate control in patients who are hypotensive.

Anticoagulation

Patients with POAF are likely at a high risk of thromboembolism considering the prothrombotic state in the post operative period. Though there no guidelines regarding anti-coagulation for post cardiac surgery AF; it is appropriate to consider anti-coagulation for patients who have POAF lasting more than 48 hours. The benefits need to be compared with the risk of anticoagulation in these patient who have had cardiac surgery.

Patients with very high risk of stroke need to be on heparin infusion until therapeutic levels of anticoagulation with coumadin are achieved. Anticoagulation should be continued for a minimum of 3 to 4 weeks.

Ventricular Tachyarrhythmia

Complex ventricular arrhythmias in the presence of coronary artery disease are a marker for more advanced anatomic disease and an independent risk factor for sudden death. Coronary artery bypass graft surgery is frequently employed to relieve angina and may improve prognosis in such patients with extensive disease. Coronary revascularization performs an anti-arrhythmic function in selected patients who have experienced previous ventricular tachycardia (VT) and/or ventricular fibrillation (VF) due to ischemia. There is, however, a subset of patients have increased incidence of ventricular arrhythmias following cardiac surgery. Ventricular arrhythmia may take the form of the benign presence of isolated premature ventricular complexes, but more importantly may predispose to the occurrence of sustained ventricular tachyarrhythmia with cardiovascular compromise. Conditions associated with ventricular arrhythmias after cardiac surgery include electrolyte abnormalities, hypoxia, ischemia, acute graft closure, reperfusion after cessation of cardiopulmonary bypass, and pro-arrhythmic effect of ionotropes and anti-arrhythmic medications.

In a observation study it was noted that complex ventricular arrhythmias [defined as Lown grades 4a (couplets), 4b (ventricular tachycardia) and 5 (R on T phenomenon)] as documented by pre-discharge 24 hour ambulatory electrocardiographic monitoring occurred in 57% of cardiac surgery patients. 43 % of patients had no or simple ventricular arrhythmias (Lown grades 1 to 3). Risk factors analyzed included age, sex, diabetes, hypertension, smoking, preoperative digoxin or propranolol therapy, cardiopulmonary bypass time, aortic cross- clamp time, number of vessels bypassed, peak creatine kinase (CK) elevation and pericarditis. No risk factor identified patients at higher risk for complex ventricular arrhythmias. Patients were followed up for 6 to 24 months (mean 16). Patients with complex ventricular arrhythmias did not have a higher incidence of sudden death, cardiac death, syncope, angina, myocardial infarction or cerebro-vascular accident (Rubin, Nieminski et al. 1985). In another study frequent complex ventricular ectopies in patients with reduced left ventricular ejection fraction of less than 40% was associated with 33% incidence of sudden death at an average follow-up of 15 months. Patients with normal left ventricular function had no worsening of their outcome (Huikuri, Yli-Mayry et al. 1990). Patients with sustained ventricular tachycardia on the other hand have a poor short and long term outcome with only 50% inpatient survival rate (Smith, Leung et al. 1992). Aggressive management with correction of reversible causes need to be considered. Electrophysiologic study and implantable cardioverter-defibrillator needs to be considered in patients with recurrent sustained ventricular tachycardia. Close attention to identification and treatment of electrolytes, ischemia, or mechanical complications of surgery.

In the CAST trial suppression of these ventricular ectopics/premature beats following cardiac ischemia were associated with poor outcome. The medications studies in these trials include Flecanide, Encanide and sotalol (Echt, Liebson et al. 1991; Waldo, Camm et al.

1996). Experience with these medications in ischemic setting could be extrapolated to cardiac surgery patients.

Electrical defibrillation or cardioversion needs to be performed for patients with hemodynamically unstable ventricular tachycardia or ventricular fibrillation. A energy level of 200 J biphasic is considered just like in the management of non-surgical patients. In patients who are hemodynamically stable but have persistent sustained tachycardia, medication including Lidocaine (1 – 1.5 mg/kg followed by infusion at 1 – 4 mg/min) or Procainamide (20-50 mg/min loading followed by 1 – 4 mg/min) or Amiodarone (150 mg bolus over 10 mins, followed by 1 mg/min) need to be considered. In patients with slow ventricular tachycardia, overdrive pacing could be considered if ventricular epicardial pacing wires are still in place.

Bradyarrhythmias

About 1% of patients undergoing coronary bypass graft surgery and 6-8% of patients undergoing valvular surgery required permanent pacemaker (PPM) implantation after the surgery for bradycardia or atrioventricular (AV) block (Goldman, Hill et al. 1984; Keefe, Griffin et al. 1985; Caspi, Amar et al. 1989). About 20,000 PPM are implanted each year in the United States for post surgical bradycardia, given the fact that about 500,000 CABG and 200,000 valve surgeries are performed annually (Lloyd-Jones, Adams et al. 2010). Risk factors for requiring PPM include advanced age, preexisting cardiac conduction system disease, prolonged cardiopulmonary bypass time (CPBT), and valvular surgery (Meimoun, Zeghdi et al. 2002). The risk prediction score developed to assess for requirement of PPM in the post operative period; assigns 2 points to right bundle branch block, multi-valvular surgery and 1 point each to age >75 yrs, PR interval >200ms, left bundle branch, prior history of valvular surgery and multi-valvular surgery not including tricuspid valve (Koplan, Stevenson et al. 2003).

The AV node lies in close proximity to the non-coronary cusp of the aortic valve and the commissure between the non and the right coronary sinus. It lies between the posterior-medial commissure of the anterior leaflet of the mitral valve and the septal leaflet of the tricuspid valve. Risk of conduction abnormalities increases with aggressive debridement of mitral annular tissue, placement of deep sutures, and impingement of the prosthetic ring on conduction tissue. Local edema from injury to the adjacent tissue could also result in temporary conduction system disturbances. Ischemic injury to cardiac conduction system, reflected by CPBT and the choice of cardioplegic solution, has also been noted to be associated with requirement of PPM. Sinus node could be injured in cases of biatrial incisions which is performed to provide adequate exposure of the mitral and tricuspid valves (Utley, Leyland et al. 1995). Interrupted sutures (vs continuous) and stentless valves (vs stented) reduce the events of conduction tissue abnormalities (Totaro, Calamai et al. 2000; Elahi and Usmaan 2006). Recent advances in non-surgical replacement of the aortic valve with percutaneous aortic valve implantation has also been associated with a need for PPM in up to 30% of cases (Piazza, Onuma et al. 2008).

Resolution of edema, reduction in inflammation of the tissue and improved blood flow to the AV node is suggested to improve conduction in the days following cardiac surgery. Although longterm recovery is possible, patients with symptomatic bradycardia, junctional or accelerated idioventricular escape rhythm, or those with intermittent AV nodal conduction may required PPM placed and may result in symptom relief with PPM. Thus, from a practical point of view, American College of Cardiology/American Heart Association/Heart Rhythm Society device-based therapy guidelines assigns a class I recommendation to PPM implantation in patients who postoperatively develop complete or high-degree AV block that is unlikely to resolve by 7 days (Epstein, DiMarco et al. 2008).

Conclusion

Arrhythmias are common following cardiac surgeries. A close monitoring in the perioperative period helps in early detection and management of these arrhythmias in these patients. Patients with higher risk of post operative atrial fibrillation need to identified before surgery and need to considered for prophylactic management. Older patients undergoing multivalvular surgery are at a higher risk of bradycardia in the postoperative period and have higher likelihood of requring permanent pacemaker implantation.

References

Aranki, S. F., D. P. Shaw, et al. (1996). "Predictors of atrial fibrillation after coronary artery surgery. Current trends and impact on hospital resources." *Circulation* 94(3): 390-397.

Blommaert, D., M. Gonzalez, et al. (2000). "Effective prevention of atrial fibrillation by continuous atrial overdrive pacing after coronary artery bypass surgery." *J. Am. Coll Cardiol.* 35(6): 1411-1415.

Burgess, D. C., M. J. Kilborn, et al. (2006). "Interventions for prevention of post-operative atrial fibrillation and its complications after cardiac surgery: a meta-analysis." *Eur. Heart J.* 27(23): 2846-2857.

Caspi, J., R. Amar, et al. (1989). "Frequency and significance of complete atrioventricular block after coronary artery bypass grafting." *Am. J. Cardiol.* 63(9): 526-529.

Cavolli, R., K. Kaya, et al. (2008). "Does sodium nitroprusside decrease the incidence of atrial fibrillation after myocardial revascularization?: a pilot study." *Circulation* 118(5): 476-481.

Crystal, E., S. J. Connolly, et al. (2002). "Interventions on prevention of postoperative atrial fibrillation in patients undergoing heart surgery: a meta-analysis." *Circulation* 106(1): 75-80.

Daoud, E. G., S. A. Strickberger, et al. (1997). "Preoperative amiodarone as prophylaxis against atrial fibrillation after heart surgery." *N. Engl. J. Med.* 337(25): 1785-1791.

Eagle, K. A., R. A. Guyton, et al. (1999). "ACC/AHA Guidelines for Coronary Artery Bypass Graft Surgery: A Report of the American College of Cardiology/American Heart Association Task Force on Practice Guidelines (Committee to Revise the 1991

Guidelines for Coronary Artery Bypass Graft Surgery). American College of Cardiology/American Heart Association." *J. Am. Coll Cardiol.* 34(4): 1262-1347.

Echt, D. S., P. R. Liebson, et al. (1991). "Mortality and morbidity in patients receiving encainide, flecainide, or placebo. The Cardiac Arrhythmia Suppression Trial." *N. Engl. J. Med.* 324(12): 781-788.

Elahi, M. and K. Usmaan (2006). "The bioprosthesis type and size influence the postoperative incidence of permanent pacemaker implantation in patients undergoing aortic valve surgery." *J. Interv. Card Electrophysiol.* 15(2): 113-118.

Epstein, A. E., J. P. DiMarco, et al. (2008). "ACC/AHA/HRS 2008 Guidelines for Device-Based Therapy of Cardiac Rhythm Abnormalities: a report of the American College of Cardiology/American Heart Association Task Force on Practice Guidelines (Writing Committee to Revise the ACC/AHA/NASPE 2002 Guideline Update for Implantation of Cardiac Pacemakers and Antiarrhythmia Devices): developed in collaboration with the American Association for Thoracic Surgery and Society of Thoracic Surgeons." *Circulation* 117(21): e350-408.

Fuster, V., L. E. Ryden, et al. (2006). "ACC/AHA/ESC 2006 Guidelines for the Management of Patients with Atrial Fibrillation: a report of the American College of Cardiology/American Heart Association Task Force on Practice Guidelines and the European Society of Cardiology Committee for Practice Guidelines (Writing Committee to Revise the 2001 Guidelines for the Management of Patients With Atrial Fibrillation): developed in collaboration with the European Heart Rhythm Association and the Heart Rhythm Society." *Circulation* 114(7): e257-354.

Gibbons, R. J., K. Chatterjee, et al. (1999). "ACC/AHA/ACP-ASIM guidelines for the management of patients with chronic stable angina: executive summary and recommendations. A Report of the American College of Cardiology/American Heart Association Task Force on Practice Guidelines (Committee on Management of Patients with Chronic Stable Angina)." *Circulation* 99(21): 2829-2848.

Goldman, B. S., T. J. Hill, et al. (1984). "Permanent cardiac pacing after open-heart surgery: acquired heart disease." *Pacing Clin. Electrophysiol.* 7(3 Pt 1): 367-371.

Halonen, J., P. Loponen, et al. (2010). "Metoprolol versus amiodarone in the prevention of atrial fibrillation after cardiac surgery: a randomized trial." *Ann. Intern Med.* 153(11): 703-709.

Huikuri, H. V., S. Yli-Mayry, et al. (1990). "Prevalence and prognostic significance of complex ventricular arrhythmias after coronary arterial bypass graft surgery." *Int. J. Cardiol.* 27(3): 333-339.

Keefe, D. L., J. C. Griffin, et al. (1985). "Atrioventricular conduction abnormalities in patients undergoing isolated aortic or mitral valve replacement." *Pacing Clin. Electrophysiol.* 8(3 Pt 1): 393-398.

Koplan, B. A., W. G. Stevenson, et al. (2003). "Development and validation of a simple risk score to predict the need for permanent pacing after cardiac valve surgery." *J. Am. Coll Cardiol.* 41(5): 795-801.

Kowey, P. R., P. Dorian, et al. (2009). "Vernakalant hydrochloride for the rapid conversion of atrial fibrillation after cardiac surgery: a randomized, double-blind, placebo-controlled trial." *Circ. Arrhythm Electrophysiol.* 2(6): 652-659.

Lahey, S. J., C. T. Campos, et al. (1998). "Hospital readmission after cardiac surgery. Does "fast track" cardiac surgery result in cost saving or cost shifting?" *Circulation* 98(19 Suppl): II35-40.

Lloyd-Jones, D., R. J. Adams, et al. (2010). "Heart disease and stroke statistics--2010 update: a report from the American Heart Association." *Circulation* 121(7): e46-e215.

Mathew, J. P., R. Parks, et al. (1996). "Atrial fibrillation following coronary artery bypass graft surgery: predictors, outcomes, and resource utilization. MultiCenter Study of Perioperative Ischemia Research Group." *JAMA* 276(4): 300-306.

Meimoun, P., R. Zeghdi, et al. (2002). "Frequency, predictors, and consequences of atrioventricular block after mitral valve repair." *Am. J. Cardiol.* 89(9): 1062-1066.

Ommen, S. R., J. A. Odell, et al. (1997). "Atrial arrhythmias after cardiothoracic surgery." *N. Engl. J. Med.* 336(20): 1429-1434.

Patel, D., M. A. Gillinov, et al. (2008). "Atrial fibrillation after cardiac surgery: where are we now?" *Indian Pacing Electrophysiol. J.* 8(4): 281-291.

Piazza, N., Y. Onuma, et al. (2008). "Early and persistent intraventricular conduction abnormalities and requirements for pacemaking after percutaneous replacement of the aortic valve." *JACC Cardiovasc Interv.* 1(3): 310-316.

Rosamond, W., K. Flegal, et al. (2008). "Heart disease and stroke statistics--2008 update: a report from the American Heart Association Statistics Committee and Stroke Statistics Subcommittee." *Circulation* 117(4): e25-146.

Rubin, D. A., K. E. Nieminski, et al. (1985). "Ventricular arrhythmias after coronary artery bypass graft surgery: incidence, risk factors and long-term prognosis." *J. Am. Coll Cardiol.* 6(2): 307-310.

Smith, R. C., J. M. Leung, et al. (1992). "Ventricular dysrhythmias in patients undergoing coronary artery bypass graft surgery: incidence, characteristics, and prognostic importance. Study of Perioperative Ischemia (SPI) Research Group." *Am. Heart J.* 123(1): 73-81.

Totaro, P., G. Calamai, et al. (2000). "Continuous suture technique and impairment of the atrioventricular conduction after aortic valve replacement." *J. Card Surg.* 15(6): 418-422; discussion 423.

Utley, J. R., S. A. Leyland, et al. (1995). "Comparison of outcomes with three atrial incisions for mitral valve operations. Right lateral, superior septal, and transseptal." *J. Thorac. Cardiovasc. Surg.* 109(3): 582-587.

Waldo, A. L., A. J. Camm, et al. (1996). "Effect of d-sotalol on mortality in patients with left ventricular dysfunction after recent and remote myocardial infarction. The SWORD Investigators. Survival With Oral d-Sotalol." *Lancet* 348(9019): 7-12.

Index